DAUGHTERS
OF THE
ELDERLY

DAUGHTERS
OF THE
ELDERLY

BUILDING PARTNERSHIPS IN
CAREGIVING

Edited by

Jane Norris

INDIANA
UNIVERSITY
PRESS
Bloomington and Indianapolis

Manufactured in the United States of America

Library of Congress Cataloging-in-Publication Data

Daughters of the elderly.

Bibliography: p.
1. Parents, Aged—Care—United States.   2. Adult children—United States.   3. Daughters—United States.
I. Norris, Jane.
HV1465.D38   1988   649.8   87-46246
ISBN 0-253-31612-X
ISBN 0-253-20484-4 (pbk.)

1 2 3 4 5 92 91 90 89 88

CONTENTS

What about Sons?

The Last of Life

ACKNOWLEDGMENTS

The following are acknowledged with grateful appreciation:

Dr. Philip B. Stafford, for long-standing support of the group and all its projects; Dr. John Werner, for sustained support of the commitment to this book; Marcy Singer, for hours and hours of word processing and helpful editorial comments; Dr. George N. Lewis and Peg Petranoff, RN, for review of medical material; Gene Arnholt, for legal counsel; Jo Lawton, for leadership as nurse, mentor, caregiver, and champion of excellence in the care of the elderly; Sam Cleland, for editorial and technical assistance and the right, light, touch of humor; Mike Montgomery, Bill Meier, Dick Norris, and other family members . . . for patience and loving support.

PREFACE

To a daughter of aging parents:

This book is designed for you. What you will find on its pages are struggles very similar to your own by daughters who are your colleagues—experts very much like yourself by virtue of long practice in the art of caring and caregiving. You will also find articles by your partners—professionals who have specialized in aging or health from such fields as social work, medicine, nursing, anthropology, and law.

In times of great stress such as those brought on by the illness, injury, or impending loss of a loved one, it becomes even more difficult to analyze the problems, understand our feelings, and help make decisions regarding the care of close family, especially our parents. The book is not intended as an "answer" to these issues and responsibilities, nor is it meant to serve in any way as a substitute for professional, medical, legal, or other specific advice when you need it. Rather, it is a response from a small support group of women to an awareness of the complicated and confusing nature of the caregiving role. In this collected work we hope to help daughters identify problems and feelings and to help families talk about the issues and begin taking steps in directions that are most appropriate to each individual family.

The support group, DEBUT, for Daughters of the Elderly Bridging the Unknown Together, was organized in July 1981, sponsored by a mental health center in Indiana. The women meet weekly for discussion of the issues related to aging and caregiving and have worked consistently toward their goals, of which the primary three are: (1) non-judgmental support, (2) education in all areas of caring and coping, and (3) reaching out to others in similar circumstances.

By now you must be asking, as we are always asked, "What about sons?" Men, and indeed the whole community, either here at home or on our trips to other locations, have always been invited and encouraged to attend our educational presentations and outreach activities. The support group meetings have traditionally focused on daughters, including daughters-in-law and granddaughters, because women as nurturers, the "natural supports," most often find themselves in a caregiving role. You will see that we have included a son's personal experiences with a response about caregiving and men's issues.

The people who have written personal narratives, some anonymously, have all been associated in one way or another with the support group. The daughters, very much committed to reaching out to you, sometimes going back and forth from tears to laughter, and always in spite of reliving their own emotional pain, have shared their experiences with you, hoping to help you identify more clearly your own feelings and problems. We have learned that separation and identification of such elements in the caregiving role can help to alleviate feelings of isolation, frustration, and anxiety. Identification of feelings includes, for example, differentiating between guilt and sadness, or regret. Identification of problems includes, for example, assessing whether a loved one is suffering from a reversible, or irreversible, cause of memory loss.

The professionals address selected issues following the personal narratives, including well-being and self-care, support and advocacy for our elderly loved ones, feelings, and decision-making in health care. Their material is presented in a style and language directed not to other professionals, but to families. The articles provide information and help in sorting out the physical, mental, and emotional aspects of aging and caregiving. One of the concepts discussed, for example, is autonomy, everyone's struggle to remain "oneself" in the face of familial/societal obligations.

Provided throughout the book will be some of the educational "tools" you may need in your role, such as lists of suggested readings and some of the specialized terminology used in "aging" circles (for example, geriatrician and dementia). No attempt has been made to restrict information to given sections because the topics are obviously overlapping. The professionals have been encouraged to discuss the material in a holistic manner from the perspective of the various disciplines because we anticipate that readers will pick and choose from segments of the book. Small introductions will appear at intervals prior to sections to further acquaint you with topics or authors.

Reading parts of this book will not be easy for you. And talking it over with your families may be still more difficult. But aging is here. "What are we going to do about it?" is a question asked across the country by caregivers, families, and members of the helping professions. Perhaps what can, or must, be done is best done if we do it together.

Jane Norris

DAUGHTERS
OF THE
ELDERLY

FAMILIES AND AGING

A very small percentage (only about 5 percent) of the elderly are in long-term care institutions at any given time. The vast majority of the older adult population live independently in their communities, semi-independently with assistance from family members and community resources, or with family members who provide, or advocate for, the full range of services needed.

We begin with "Families and Aging" in recognition that families, though called "informal caregivers," are in fact *caregivers* providing services needed by family elders, sometimes twenty-four hours a day, usually without benefit of formal training or supports. "Research on families and older adults has consistently documented that families, and especially adult children, are the predominant service and health care providers to the impaired elderly" (Amy Horowitz, DSW, "Sons and Daughters as Caregivers to Older Parents: Differences in Role Performance and Consequences," Paper presented at the 34th Annual Scientific Meeting of the Gerontological Society of America, Toronto, Canada, November, 1981).

The voices of three generations of one family are heard here. Sarah, the daughter, tells the story of the events, the problems, and the feelings associated with bringing her widowed mother into her home. Karen, the granddaughter, speaks openly about her concerns for her mother and about the negative as well as the positive aspects of the situation. Carrie, the grandmother, reminisces about her life and tells what it is like for her now. Anna and Joanna, long-standing advocates for family supports, respond about generational issues as well as stress and adjustments. Dixie, who loves folklore and has recorded two volumes of it, weaves reminiscence into the pattern of our lives: useful, beneficial, significant to family relationships and tradition. Ellen's comments about normal aging and other issues in health and illness are shared with us from what may someday be her own book. She is a physician interested in holistic health care who speaks here, as in her practice, about care and prevention, sometimes to the caregiver, sometimes to the elderly.

1

EDITOR'S NOTE: The first names of the professional authors are used in these introductory remarks partly because it seems natural to do so, since they have worked with us on projects or conferences for several years, but more importantly because they are warm-hearted, dedicated, people who are as interested as you are in reducing barriers to strong effective partnerships. They had you in mind, particularly because of their years of work with older adults or caregivers, as they wrote material they hoped would help or support you.

A New Crisis

Sarah

No one ever sits down and casually, over a cup of coffee says, "I think I'll call Mother and invite her to live with me." Nor does Mother ever say, "You know, I've always wanted to live with you and your wonderful family." It is a situation that usually arises after a catastrophic event has occurred and a quick decision must be made. That is what happened to me.

My mother, aged eighty-six, came to live with me and my family on my birthday. Ironic, I thought . . . Mother coming to live with me, and fifty-two years ago today I came to live with her.

Our family had faced a series of events in recent years, events that had frequently erupted in crisis. Over the preceeding nine months Mother had been hospitalized three times for high blood pressure; Dad had been hospitalized twice for pneumonia and was admitted to a nursing home with Parkinson's Disease. Just a few months before, my sister, Linda, died of cancer after a fifteen-year struggle, and two of our four adult children were in the process of getting divorced. We were just beginning to get over the death of my father-in-law, who had passed away four years earlier of leukemia. All that, and now the doctor had called from the hospital in Mother's home town to tell me that she could no longer live alone! Our family was facing another crisis.

I could have made the trip to get Mother alone, but since I was recovering from the flu—at least I thought I was recovering—my daughter, Karen, and son, Bill decided to go with me. As luck would have it we had trouble before we started. Our car was fairly new, so we were surprised to discover that the axle had broken. We rented a car and headed for Cortland Hospital, some sixty-five miles away.

MULLING IT OVER

As we drove through the beautiful countryside my thoughts went back to that telephone call from the doctor. Mother had forgotten to take her blood pressure

3

medicine, and now another attack had sent her to the hospital. Whenever Mother forgot to take her medication her blood pressure would skyrocket, on one occasion reaching 270/125. Her forgetfulness could be fatal. The doctor said that I would have to provide full-time care. If I chose, he would make the necessary arrangements for Mother to enter a nursing home.

The doctor also told me she had short-term memory loss and apparent malnutrition. I couldn't believe it—not my mother who had always stressed good food and made the best coffee cake my family ever tasted! Impossible. But as I later started to question her it became clear that she was not eating a variety of foods. Her refrigerator revealed four dozen eggs, a tray of chicken thighs, and lunch meat. There were other foods such as butter, mayonnaise, and pickles, but it was obvious that Mother was not cooking. "Why bother cooking," she said. "It's just something to eat." She simply didn't care to eat. A decision had to be made.

The cost of nursing home care for both my parents would drain their life savings in a very short time. My mother was forgetful, but she certainly did not require the skilled care provided in an nursing home. She needed someone to keep her medicine on schedule and encourage good nutrition. She did have a bladder problem in addition to high blood pressure, but otherwise her health was fairly good. A nursing home was not necessary.

Of course Mother would come to live with us. She would be joining a family group that included my husband, Jim, myself, and our twenty-three-year-old daughter, Karen, who had just graduated from college; she was substitute-teaching while looking for full-time employment. Karen had been so helpful when Mother stayed with us last fall, and she would be very helpful in working with me in this caregiving situation.

Two of our children, Scott and Paula, lived fifty miles away, too far to be home very often. However, Bill, our oldest son, was living in the same town and would prove to be a good companion for Mother when I needed help.

I was having mixed feelings about my own career as a dental technician. Since my employer was retiring that month, my job was ending. I really wanted very much to get another job, but I was still too ill even to consider looking. Perhaps forced retirement was a blessing because coping with Mother would require a major portion of my time, at least for a while.

When we arrived at the hospital Mother was ready to leave and readily agreed to stay with us for a time.

DECEMBER

Caring for Mother has been like caring for an adult toddler. You love them deeply, you can never leave them alone, and they require constant care. They are never out of your mind. The very first month with Mother in our home has proved to be the most traumatic.

A Christmas Day visit with Dad, who was eighty-five miles away, looked impossible because of the bad weather and my continuing battle with the flu. It was bitterly cold. Temperatures hovered around zero, and the roads were icy and hazardous.

However, as things turned out, I have often felt sad and guilty because we didn't go. On Christmas morning I called the nursing home to ask them to tell Dad we would come as soon as weather conditions improved. Three days later, the doctor telephoned. Dad had just passed away. I was numb with shock. The weather was still very bad. Initial funeral arrangements were made as best I could over the telephone, including the minister, flowers, and newspaper obituary. The day before the funeral, Mother, Jim, and I drove over those icy roads and completed the funeral arrangements. I was able to take care of so many arrangements over the telephone because of the thoughtfulness of my parents. They had looked ahead to see how they might help with their future care and had given me power of attorney, made a will, bought burial plots, erected a stone, and told me what funeral home they wanted. What wonderful and caring parents.

No one ever said life would be easy, but Dad's death was simply too much for my mother, and for me. I was experiencing common family problems . . . but so many in one year? My grief and my mother's grief, as well as that of the whole family, was overwhelming, and we struggled to live one day at a time.

REFLECTIONS

We had been a very close family, living two short blocks away from my parents and four blocks from my husband's parents. My sister, who was divorced, lived with her two daughters two blocks from us. Our children were able to visit their grandparents and cousins often; we celebrated birthdays, Christmas, and Thanksgiving at our wonderful big old house. We were involved in one another's lives, caring and sharing.

When my sister remarried and moved to another part of town, we were still close because it was a small community. Two years later Jim accepted a new position in a college town sixty-five miles away, and we moved. It was during this time that Jim's father became very ill with leukemia, and we were on the road practically every weekend for eighteen months, trying to help his parents in any way we could.

My parents were in their late seventies then and still active. My father was working part-time as a school custodian, and Mother helped my sister by cooking special dishes for her when she had company—she still entertained quite often. Linda was working full-time and was very happy with her new family—she now had two teenage sons as well as her two teenage daughters.

Gradually, Dad's health deteriorated, and I began to assume more responsibility for my parents. I became their problem-solver as my father's confusion worsened. It was I who wrote the checks, took Dad to the doctor, and found a young woman to come every day to bathe, shave, and dress him. This wonderful woman also cleaned the house. But Mother needed someone at night also, and when Dad fell and cracked his pelvis, I knew that Mother could no longer care for him. He needed more care than either Mother or I could give. My sister made the necessary arrangements for Dad to enter a nursing home twenty miles from their home, adding another forty miles to my trip. Mother was terribly lonely and grieved so for Dad. It was at this time that my sister's health also declined. Linda's cancer was no longer in remission, and as she struggled with chemotherapy and frequent hospital stays, Mother had to rely more and more on herself.

Jim and I began making the 130-mile round trip every other weekend. We started very early in the morning and returned very late at night. The trip home was especially draining, both physically and emotionally. I could see all those people I loved so dearly dying a little more every time I saw them. My sister's cancer was worsening. She must have had tumors in her jaws because she was unable to get her teeth apart to open her mouth. The doctors tried very hard to correct this but were not successful; Linda lost weight and literally starved to death. She had been a dynamic person, a school nurse, loved by all the children. In addition, it had been Linda who had looked in on Mother and Dad after Jim and I moved.

That winter was especially hard for Mother and me. Mother had to sell her home—my childhood home and the last link with Linda and Dad. It was the most difficult task I have had to perform. It was just an ordinary bungalow, but it was chock-full of memories. My parents lived there forty-one years and it took several months, back and forth one day each week, to sort, sell, and give things away that meant so much to my parents. The house sold very quickly, and Mother and I had one more thing to grieve.

ALWAYS HER DAUGHTER, BUT . . .

Now Mother is living with us. We are her family and she is ours. It is not an easy job being a caregiver, and I struggle to meet the demands of this confused woman. I am not a nurse, and yet now I must know about diseases I have heard of only recently. My mother complained a fews weeks ago that something was wrong with her mind . . . she didn't know what, but she was dizzy, confused, and knew that her mind was not right. About a week later her blood pressure dropped to 90/50, and the doctor decided to cut in half the dosage of her medicine for high blood pressure. After that she felt better. Her medication dosage had been too high.

Mother had a chronic bladder problem. She was incontinent but had tried to take care of her problem the best she could. She would tell me that, yes, it was a problem, but all old people get that way. I believed her. I didn't know about that sort of thing, but I decided that she should see a urologist—Mother was distraught and my home was beginning to smell. Mother was so embarrassed about her incontinence that she would sit only on her leather chair in the living room.

After examining Mother, the urologist said she was brimming with infection, even though she had never complained of pain. He suspected that her anti-depressant medicine was causing much of the problem. Mother did get over the bladder infection, but the doctor was concerned and did not dismiss her. He repeatedly told her that she could regain control of her bladder. After consulting with Mother's cardiologist, he discontinued the antidepressant medicine, and her irritated bladder began to heal. The urologist told Mother that healing would take weeks. Now, eight weeks later, she is beginning to have feeling in her bladder and has stopped wetting the bed. No longer incontinent, she can wear slacks, and that solved another problem—being cold.

Mother never wore slacks until recently—she always wore dresses. Because she complained about being cold, I bought slacks for her and very gently suggested that she wear them. She told me in no uncertain terms that she would never wear slacks. They reminded her of pajamas, and I could just take them back. I didn't take them back, and finally she told me that since I was going to make her wear them anyway she guessed she would try them. Now she wears slacks all the time. She loves them—everyone comments about how nice she looks, and she just beams. I have quit expecting Mother to cooperate readily. I just do what I think should be done. This has been very hard for me because in situations like this I become my mother's "mother." I keep switching roles all day—daughter one time, "mother" another—and never, never can I get used to Mother's confusion. She thought all those young people were my husband's children by his first wife. (My husband has never been married before.) I told her, "Mother, you have me mixed up with my sister." That didn't satisfy her, and I had to rehash my whole marriage—"all those kids are mine." Confusion is hard to live with, but it is something I have had to learn to adjust to and be very patient about.

We have tried to make Mother's adjustment to living with us as smooth as we can. Mother did not want to live with us. She told me over and over that she wanted to live in her house at 204 E. Elm Street. She had friends, she said, and she was not lonely. But the doctor was firm; she could not live alone. We moved her bedroom furniture into her new bedroom, and we thought that with her TV and rocking chair she would be comfortable. She has her own bathroom next to the bedroom, and we assumed that she would enjoy the quiet and privacy whenever she wanted to get away from the family . . . *not so.* This same lady who told me a year ago she was never lonely cannot bear to have me out of her sight, ever. She does not want to be alone.

This morning, as I made out the monthly budget and wrote the utility checks, my mother came into the room and announced that she was lonely and just wanted to sit with me. The cat was lonely also and decided to "help." Even as I write this chapter of my life, at the kitchen table, I am constantly interrupted with

"What are you writing?" I quickly cover the paper and answer, "Oh, nothing." I feel like a schoolgirl caught writing a note in class.

LIGHT AT THE END OF THE TUNNEL

Because I was beginning to fall apart, I decided that Mother and I needed help. I saw an article about a support group in the newspaper and my daughter, Karen, called the sponsors of the group, for all the necessary information about meetings and so on.

My daughter and I both joined the group and my husband stays with Mother while Karen and I attend the weekly meeting. It is good to be away from home and to socialize with new friends. I was beginning to feel very isolated, and I know my family was concerned. That first meeting was a source of information, information, information. Others in the group had had similar problems, and they gave me suggestions and ideas about how to care for Mother. My friends said that Mother needed to get out, have some fun, go out to lunch once a week . . . a simple idea but one that had not occurred to me. Mother now has her hair shampooed and set every week, and we go out to lunch. We enjoy this outing, and it helps Mother to learn about her new town. She is also just beginning to go to church again.

Feelings of depression and grieving cannot be put on the back burner and expected to go away. In the last few weeks, when we are alone, I have begun having conversations with Mother concerning our feelings over the loss of our husband/father and daughter/sister. I believe this has helped us as we cry and share memories. My mother doesn't talk much, and my talking about our good times and sad times seems to help us accept our losses. Not only has death been with us all but also, for her, the loss of home and familiar surroundings, church, and friends.

Mother was not an educated woman. She worked in a factory most of her life. She never had time for fun things. Her hobby, sewing, was a necessity. She made all her clothes and all my sister's and my clothes until we were in high school. Later, she made clothes for her granddaughters. She never belonged to clubs, didn't read much, and now she finds too much time on her hands. She can no longer sew very well and cannot make sense out of watching TV. But she wants to be part of the family, and so she sits with us while we watch television.

ELDERHOUSE

Mother has been going to Elderhouse, an adult day care program, every Friday afternoon. She looks forward to this day because it is on Fridays that outings take place. The participants go to parks, take drives in the country, go to quilt fairs or to anything that might be interesting to the folks. Mother loves this and tells me about the picnic she had and about the trip. It is especially nice in the fall. I enjoy the three hours of doing whatever I like, knowing that Mother is in good hands.

My friends in the support group have been concerned about me and have suggested that I spend some time having fun—maybe a movie or dinner out with my husband. I feel guilty leaving my mother (of course someone is staying with her), but I know it is good for me.

Our whole family has changed since Mother has come to live with us. Three of my adult children do not live at home, but they stop by frequently and stay with Mother whenever they can. Karen is a great help and sometimes can get Mother to do something that she refused to do when I asked. All of us are more sensitive to the needs of the elderly, and we all work together to help Grandma help herself and find some happiness. My husband takes us for rides in the country or to the lake and cares for Mother so I can shop or go to the library. He has tried to make her feel wanted and a part of this family.

Mother tries to keep busy doing hand-sewing, a limited amount of food preparation, or straightening her room, but more and more she naps. She likes an orderly house—it's less confusing to her—and she likes the house to be quiet. She becomes very confused if our normal routine is changed, and she is usually disoriented when first arising in the morning or right after a nap. She enjoys our two cats, and sometimes her only exercise is letting Smokey and Sparky in and out of the house.

It sometimes is difficult to care for Mother. I try to keep my sense of humor, and I try to find time to do things that make me feel good. After all, who will take care of Mother if I wear myself out and become ill?

I feel a sense of pride and satisfaction as a caregiver. In later years I want to look back and know in my heart that I tried to make the last years of my mother's life as happy and as comfortable as I could.

Grandma Came to Live with Us

Karen

Grandma came to live with us after her doctor said she could no longer live alone; she wasn't able to meet her own basic needs. I knew it would be difficult adjusting to having a "new" family member, but I had no idea of what a long, draining, frustrating experience it would be. In the end, yes, there are rewards. But first there is frustration, guilt, and anger.

Grandma was raised to believe you should work hard, save every penny, keep your home spotless, and go to church on Sunday. She found conversation around the dinner table to be a waste of time better spent doing dishes. She was angry that Mom wasn't constantly cleaning the house and preparing elaborate meals. She couldn't understand how important private time was to each of us and would walk into any room, without knocking, and demand to know what we were doing. This was a stressful time for all of us as we tried to accommodate Grandma without giving up the things that were really important to our home atmosphere.

Bringing Grandma home to live with us was especially difficult for Mom. I watched her grapple with the day-to-day role struggle between her and Grandma. One moment she was "daughter," the next moment, "mother." Always, she was confused and dissatisfied with the lack of definition as to how she should interact with Grandma. I watched Mom be manipulated by Grandma and saw how overwhelmed with guilt she constantly felt since nothing she did ever seemed to make Grandma happy. I watched Mom grow more tired day by day because her nights were spent worrying about Grandma. I saw her withdraw from the world, not knowing or caring about world events or everyday chit chat. Grandma—her care, her problems, her life—became the sole focus of Mom's attention. Mother cried frequently, was easily upset, and became rather absent-minded. She was not getting out at all and had no one to talk to that could relate to her problems. I became quite concerned for both her physical and mental health.

During this time I felt very helpless and ineffective. I couldn't stand to see my mother manipulated by Grandma, yet I knew she had to work things out with Grandma on her own without any intervention. I loved my grandmother and knew that she wasn't aware of how some of her behavior was affecting Mom. Still, I found myself becoming my mother's defender—doing what I could to keep Grandma from picking on Mom (as I saw it).

This time period was spotted with medical crises. Grandma's blood pressure would alternately skyrocket and plummet, and we would have to rush her to the doctor's office or hospital. Getting her blood pressure under control with a minimal amount of drug intervention took time, trial, and error. In addition, like many elderly people, Grandma had multiple health problems requiring several medications—each a different dosage, each with its own set of side effects. Organizing and monitoring her medication has been an education in itself.

Grandma went through many periods of being homesick. She couldn't understand why she could no longer live alone in her own home. We felt terribly guilty because the best we could do was to tell her that her doctor felt she would be better off living in our home. Somehow, this never seemed like an adequate answer.

Also during this time period, Grandpa died after an extended stay at a nursing home. We had barely recovered from the death of my aunt, my mother's sister, nine months earlier. All this grief weighed on the whole family—particularly Grandma and Mom.

As time passed, however, things improved. We've been able to come to terms with our grief and have successfully adjusted to having Grandma here with us. Grandma has accepted our home as her home and has even gone out into the community and made some friends.

Having Grandma in our home has taught me so many things. I have become more patient with other people and more understanding and appreciative of other people's viewpoints. I have learned that lowering my expectations of how a person should behave (in this case, my grandmother) doesn't mean I'm adopting a defeatist attitude; I know that realistically there will always be ambiguities and "gray areas." Because of this I can accept and appreciate Grandma for what she is now, not what she used to be or what I wish she would be.

Everyone in our family has become more comfortable about communicating with the elderly, thanks to Grandma. We understand now that elderly people are all individuals and that there is no uniform way to deal with them. Too often people make the mistake of thinking that all the elderly should be dealt with in all situations as if they were children; we've learned the strength and value of flexibility. For instance, Mom frequently asks Grandma to help out in the kitchen. I used to cringe at this activity because I thought Grandma wasn't able to help prepare a meal without constant supervision. I was wrong. Grandma enjoys working in the kitchen. It makes her feel she's really a part of the family. Treating her as if she were a child, unable to help out, would only have hurt her and kept her from from accepting our home as her home.

Having Grandma in our house has brought me closer to my mother and forced me to see her in a different light. Mother is a daughter to a woman, too, just like me, but I had never understood the force of this relationship in her life until now. I see my mother more as a person now, not just my mom, because I've seen her in the vulnerable role of child. I've learned that she isn't invincible, and I've become more understanding of her need to come to grips with issues at her own pace, not the pace that I would impose on her. I'm accepting the fact that there are certain battles that I can't fight for Mom, and in learning this I've taken some of the pressure off of her to conform to a rigid mother-role. I hope I'm helping her to experience and react to Grandma in her own way. I want Mom to know that I love her even when she appears vulnerable, even when she isn't in 100 percent control.

I have developed an awareness of and sensitivity toward all issues relating to the elderly and feel an instant rapport with anyone I meet who has an elderly person in their life and is struggling with that relationship. I've grown impatient and even angry with grandchildren who are oblivious to the powerful feelings and issues developing between their parents and grandparents as they age. Too often they merely shake their heads at what they view as a tendency on the part of the mother to overreact to things when it comes to dealing with the grandparents. Most grandchildren don't understand how much pitching in and helping out with the care of a grandparent could mean to their mother. They don't know that the comfort and validation that they can give to their mothers can do wonders for both of them and bring them much closer, too. I've met young people who are involved in caring for one or more grandparents and have felt a deep respect for them. I know that they are very special, giving, caring people and that they love their families enough to be there when they're needed, to give back some of what they've received from their parents and grandparents over the years.

Having Grandma in our home has forced me to face many of the big issues that affect a person's whole life. I've learned how important it is to value every minute and to live life to its fullest, always. I've learned how important it is to develop many interests, since you never know when you may have to give up some activity that has been of great value to you. Having many interests means that should I ever have to give up something, I'll have other activities to fill the void.

I have learned what depression really is. Therefore, I am more positive about my own life because I am not so quick to label problems as a result of "the blues." I have seen both my mother and grandmother depressed to the point of physical and mental immobilization, coping with grief and changing roles. I know that this is a serious ailment, which should be taken seriously by the whole family—not just brushed off as a meaningless, ordinary occurrence.

I've done quite a bit of thinking about death and dying, and while I haven't come to any conclusions about these issues, I'm grateful that I'm thinking about them when I'm twenty-four instead of avoiding these thoughts until I must face the reality of my own death. I think that one of the reasons people are uncomfortable around the elderly is because of their own fears of aging, dying, and death—yet we have so much to learn from these people who have traveled so far and must now look back over their lives and try to come to terms with themselves. My grandmother is generally healthy, and yet I know that because of her age (eighty-six), she feels a need to reach some sort of peace with herself since she feels faced with her own mortality. As she reminisces, she often says things that make me believe she is trying to bring closure to some of the major events in her life. She talks about selling her home, about how she felt about the house. Her home was very important to her; she had lived there for over forty years and had raised her children there. She didn't want to sell it but she'd adjusted to the fact that she couldn't take care of it anymore; the house had become a burden. Now she can look back on the whole experience and say that it was a good thing to sell the house. She has tied up some important emotional loose ends.

We tend to avoid thinking about death, but I know that being involved in the care of all my grandparents has helped me to accept death as a part of life; in that acceptance I can let go of the fear of dying and use that energy to do what I can to find meaning and happiness, instead of wasting it in fear. I don't know of any person better able to teach this lesson to a young person than a grandparent.

I've learned that it is crucial to take responsibility for our own health and that this becomes even more important as we age. We need to become partners with our doctors in our health care. Through my grandmother's experiences with doctors, I'm learning how important it is to communicate my health needs and to practice preventive health care. Perhaps this will help me to avoid in my old age some of the ailments I see my grandma dealing with now.

Part of what determines our health in later years is our attitudes and feelings about what old age should be like. My grandmother feels that she has earned the right through a lifetime of hard work to spend her later years just sitting in a big, comfortable chair. Yet it concerns me that this kind of behavior might be harmful to her health since it keeps her body from getting even a minimal amount of exercise. Also, the more we ignore our own health needs as we age, the more this responsibility falls onto the shoulders of the caregiver. It is very scary and stressful to be responsible for someone else's body. I've seen this happen to my mother and grandmother. At the doctor's office my grandmother sits mute— refusing to communicate with the doctor because she's never known how to talk to a doctor and feels too uncomfortable attempting to do so now when she's eighty-six. My mother does her best to guess at what is bothering my grandmother, but there is always that scary possibility of being wrong.

I've also learned there is no sense in the idea of keeping this kind of problem within the family—especially when the family doesn't know how to deal with it.

It is not a sign of weakness to reach out for help; rather, it is a sign of strength to recognize your limits and seek out help so that you don't burn yourself out. This is what brought my mother and me to the support group. We were growing weaker. We were tired. We were confused and running out of ideas. We were losing our ability to cope.

The group has given us strength. We have people to talk to who are going through similar situations, and we have a source of information to educate ourselves about caring for the elderly. We learned about the Adult Day Care Program through the group, and this has given Grandma an outlet—an opportunity to meet other people and get out into the community. Sharing our experiences with others has turned a crisis into a manageable situation.

Bringing Grandma to live with our family was another milestone of life, like getting married or having children. It's a struggle at first, and somewhat of a shock. But once you're through the initial adjustment period, you look back and realize that although you made mistakes, you still made it through. You've weathered the storm, now it's calmer, and you know you could do it again if you had to. Mom no longer stays awake at night worrying about Grandma. Oh, yes, there are still some sleepless nights, but mostly things are okay.

Grandma is part of our family now. She's not some distant relative we see only occasionally, but an everyday part of our lives. We see her strengths and weaknesses and share her good days and bad. We witness her aging and find affirmation for our own.

We've been tested. At a time when Mom and Dad were anticipating being a two-member family again and when my siblings and I were ready to jump into the responsibility and excitement of young adulthood, we brought another person into our family. The timing couldn't have been worse, but the outcome couldn't have been better. We've managed to become a new family, and that in and of itself is a comfort.

The Caregiving Family

Anna H. Zimmer
M. Joanna Mellor

Karen and Sarah give us a moving account of their family's experience in adjusting to a series of demanding changes. Their story can best be understood by looking at the developmental tasks and family dynamics, first in a general way and then as specific to this situation. This should be done from the perspective of the three generations involved as well as from the total family context.[1]

THE OLDER GENERATION—THE GRANDPARENT

The major struggle for the oldest generation is adjusting to an onslaught of losses.[2] This may be loss of spouse, change in residence which can include giving up the "old homestead" and a move to shared quarters, loss of status in no longer being the head of a household, the physical losses of various bodily functions, economic changes, losses of old friends and social interaction, or financial reverses and adjustments. Aging brings with it the task of accepting dependency in a variety of areas and of replacing some of life's satisfactions with others.

Anna H. Zimmer, MSW, social worker and lecturer, has over thirty years experience working with the aged and their families. Formerly director of the Natural Supports Program that developed the earliest models of community-based caregiver support groups, she is currently director of Media Assistance to Caregivers at the Brookdale Center on Aging at Hunter College. Videotapes related to support groups and caregiver coping will be available from this program.

M. Joanna Mellor, MS, is coordinator of the Hunter College/Mt. Sinai Geriatric Education Center, N.Y. She was formerly program analyst with the National Supports Program Community Service Society, N.Y., and project assistant, Third Age Center, Fordham University.

The grandmother now living in her daughter's home may become depressed by these losses or may slowly take on the role of sharing the family history—remembering old recipes and holiday traditions even though she may no longer do the cooking and preparations. For many of today's aged there is also the need to adjust to a whole different set of values related to sexual norms, marriage and divorce, money management, and the tremendous revolution in media and technology. Utilizing resources, whether they are related to medical services or the senior center, entitlements or purchased services, also requires a set of new skills. Sharing emotional pain through grieving and accepting the support of another generation is still another task for this oldest generation.

THE MIDDLE GENERATION—THE ADULT CHILD

Providing care for the older, parent generation generally occurs at the least advantageous time for the middle generation. This may be the stage when adult children are looking toward their own impending retirement, adjusting to the empty nest as their own children leave home. Perhaps, for the middle-aged women, it is a time for re-entry into the work world and for facing their own aging and possible physical deficits. For women this is an especially demanding time of life, as they have traditionally carried most of the burden of caregiving for the aged. For women in this position there is a struggle to balance the needs of their aging relatives, their own children, and possibly of their own grandchildren, being wife, mother, and daughter simultaneously. All of this may be happening just as they had hoped to find some time to "be one's own person."[3]

Research has shown that families do care and take responsibility whatever the quality of the earlier relationship to those aged. However, there may also be a reactivation of old unresolved conflicts with the older parent and/or with the siblings with whom parent care plans are being made. Then the stress of coping with caregiving becomes more acute and more difficult to resolve.[4]

More recently, some families are faced with the additional task of responsibility for their recently divorced children and grandchildren. Perhaps these demands include "moving back home" and further competition for the space an older parent might claim. Setting priorities for the use of the middle generation's resources, both emotional and concrete, becomes a focal point for adjustment. Clearly it is this middle or "sandwich" generation that has one of the most complicated tasks to handle.

THE YOUNGER GENERATION—THE GRANDCHILD

The younger generation, grandchildren, may be at various stages of development when the grandparent requires care. Perhaps they have just left college with its attendant adjustment problems or they may be recently married, divorced, or single parents. They may be adapting to the demands of a beginning career or advanced education. In all of these transitions into independent adulthood there is the growth of the individual self, the emancipation from their own parents, and then the onset of responsibilities for either their aging parents and/or grandparents. Just as the middle generation has to set priorities, so does this younger group of grandchildren. Whether the demands of the grandparents are for "hands on" care, emotional support, holiday involvement, or daily contact, there is a need to sort out what each person can contribute. The younger generation of today may be more mobile than those in past years but seems to be just as interested in knowing its family roots and hence turns to its grandparents for this history. Thus, there is a continued reciprocity that can take place and ease tensions.

To be noted, too, is the impact on the younger generation of the recognition of the toll caregiving may take of their parents or of the satisfaction gained. This can provide a role model for the future.

Our understanding of the dynamics of the caregiving family is further enhanced if we understand at just what stage each generation described above finds itself. Clarifying the stages of development within the family setting gives us a framework for assessing the potentials for stress, the kind of strengths the family can draw upon, the services needed, and the possibility of arriving at the optimal level of functioning for family members.

SARAH—THE DAUGHTER'S STORY

Sarah's story is both universal and unique. It is universal in that it is common for an adult daughter to assume responsibility for a mother as she becomes frail, and unique in that every situation is special, shaped by the nuances and personalities of the principal actors and their past and present history. Sarah and her mother are no exception.

In spite of the universality of the situation, the decision of adult children to take an aging parent into their homes to live with them is nearly always a decision that is made under crisis conditions. The decision is made under pressure characterized by an urgency and an immediacy that precludes planning. Sarah receives the doctor's phone call and makes the trip to bring Mother back to her home. Given time to plan, Sarah, her mother, and Sarah's own family would probably still decide upon this course of action, but in making the decision under the pressure of time, there is no opportunity for emotional adjustment or preparation. The progression from caring at a distance to providing care within the home is determined by the increasing needs of Sarah's mother which cannot be diverted or forestalled, but the decision to take Mother under one's roof is still made at a point of crisis.

The suddenness is apparent in Sarah's story although she is no stranger to the pain and stress of caring for a family member. She tells us that over a period of a few years, one by one of the closeknit and caring family suffer their own traumas, so that not only does the total amount of needed care in this family increase, but fewer family members are available to provide the care. Sarah finds herself with the responsibility for shouldering the caring burden and making decisions. Her mother's physical crisis demands that Sarah make reasoned decisions and execute plans even as she is in the midst of mourning her father's accelerating frailty and the loss of her sister while also fulfilling the role of wife and mother to her own children.

Events occur and Sarah's life is shaped by them. A halt is placed on Sarah's own plans to find a new job after the retirement of her employer. A decision to work part-time or to opt for an early retirement appears to be frequently linked to the need to provide care for a frail parent or spouse.

Just as a new parent learns to care for an infant, Sarah must become an expert in parent care overnight. Sarah is faced with the necessity to recognize the signs that presage medical emergencies and to understand the side effects of medications. The health professions are changing in this regard, but too few doctors are trained in the care of the geriatric patient, and too little is known of the interaction of various drugs and medications to allow for unquestioning acceptance of physician's directives. The mother's confusion resulting from an overmedication for high blood pressure and the connection between her antidepressant prescription and her bladder infection are sadly not uncommon. Sarah, like all such caregiving daughters, learns to become vigilant.

Sarah's story is the narrative of how her daily life has been changed by the decision to take her mother into her home. In spite of the difficulties and tensions that this creates, Sarah never suggests that this was an unwelcome or regretted decision. Sarah and her mother are members of a loving, caring family in which concern for each other and closeness has always been the norm. Such a family history can make it difficult to acknowledge the pressures of providing care. How can caring for a loved one be a burden? And if it is, can a dutiful and genuinely loving daughter be permitted to express this? It *is* possible to acknowledge the drawbacks and tensions inherent in a situation without regretting the underlying decision that creates the situation. It is clear from Sarah's story that there has been and still remains much love and sensitivity between mother and daughter, and perhaps it is just because of this continuing love and sensitivity that the burden of caring is so great. Recognizing the pressures involved in providing such care does not mean that one is an unloving child. This is not to suggest, however, that taking a frail parent into one's own home is the only right choice or that that choice, once made, cannot be modified. Each family, each elderly parent, each son or daughter must determine what is right for their own family and themselves.

KAREN—THE GRANDDAUGHTER'S STORY

Karen, the young adult grandchild, clearly describes the complicated interactions of the multi-generational household as the family deals with the crisis in the life of its oldest member. Her responsibility for the disabled elder is not an isolated response but is related to where she is in her own life development, as part of the overall family stage and then in the family as it is reformed when Grandma comes to live with them.

Some of the central issues revolve around each generation's set of values. How does one use time and space? What are the expectations in each family for and from each generation?[5] How does Karen feel as she sees her mother respond to the stress of caring for the grandmother? Is there resentment, understanding, empathy, sharing, guilt, conflict, satisfaction, or exchange? Karen clearly identifies each of these emotions and shares the process that occurs in the adjustment to caregiving.

Karen's story identifies the different stages of family response to stress in coping. The initial frustration, guilt, and anger are seen from her vantage point. Frustration and anger are related to the elder's intrusion on the nuclear family— in this case one in which Karen is making her own way in her own professional life while continuing as an integral part of the household and family. The homeostasis of the family is affected by her relationship to her grandmother as well as to her mother and father.

STRESS AND ADJUSTMENT

The stresses of caring for an older, frail person in your own home are legion and are noted here by both Sarah and Karen. Stress is felt in both concrete and emotional terms.[6]

Initially there are practical concerns connected with the level and type of care needed. How much should be done for the older person, how much should the older person be encouraged to do for him/herself? What about level of medication or diet? Few families are knowledgeable in these areas but, when providing care for an older person, are faced with questions that demand immediate solutions. A feeling of inadequacy or of being out of control is often the consequence until the needed skill and knowledge are learned.

The demand for constant attention as described by Sarah is time consuming and intrudes on the caregiver's privacy and sense of self as an individual with her/his own needs. Karen mentions the lack of "private time." Ironically, the constant demands, whether verbalized or not, create feelings of isolation in the caregiver.

Caring for a loved family member automatically brings to the fore emotions and feelings connected to the family life. Sarah has to redefine her role in relationship to her mother and, having done this, has to come to terms with the adjusted role.

After the initial recognition of the negative aspects of their new roles, each generation seems able to begin to deal with the stress—in practical terms and in handling emotional reactions. A certain amount of compromise appears to take place as resources are identified and utilized for a variety of needs. Only then do the more positive aspects of this new role begin to emerge. It is clear that each generation is going through the filial crisis at their own pace—arriving at filial maturity and thus being able to free themselves to handle the inevitable stress of the aging dependent grandmother.

New relationships are formed within the family setting and create a readjustment of all other family relationships as the status quo shifts and a new equilibrium is sought. Not all families are or can be as understanding and supportive as the one portrayed here. Other emotional or physical demands on a family may be occurring simultaneously and may delay or prevent readjustments and realignments.

NEEDED ADJUSTMENTS

When an elderly parent gives up his/her own home and moves into the home of an adult child, a variety of adjustments and actions occur.

The easiest adjustments to effect are the concrete, practical ones. The rearrangement of furniture, the additional place setting at the dinner table, the alteration of family living patterns to include the extra person, all fall within this category. While the family that opens its home to an older person feels these adjustments, it is the older person who is experiencing the greatest adjustment by changing her/his total surroundings and patterns of day-to-day living.

The tasks of the relocated elder must be examined. It is the older person who relinquishes most in terms of familiar surroundings, a neighborhood, and friends. Sarah and Karen both mention how they have consciously helped Sarah's mother build new contacts and new interests to replace those that were left behind. Attendance at the senior club, weekly lunch outings, drives into the countryside, and church attendance all combine to provide Sarah's mother with new interests and patterns to mark her days.

Activities through which the older person can be a contributing family member are of importance. Sarah's mother helps out in the kitchen, sews occasionally, and lets the cats in and out. These chores may not seem of immense consequence but confirm Sarah's mother as a participating family member. In the past there had always been an exchange of assistance between the generations, and though the level of exchange may now be uneven, Sarah's mother can still contribute and does so. The nature of assistance given by the older person will vary depending on his/her ability, but with imagination and creativity ways can be found for even the very frail and bedbound to contribute to the special nature of his/her family life.

The mother/grandmother is trying to achieve what might be termed parental maturity, by allowing her relatives to be her advocates in medical planning and compliance with medications, by locating resources that she can then utilize, by handling her own struggle with independence and dependence. As she arrives at this point she seems more capable of sharing the family history, becoming a role model for the younger generation who see her as surviving many crises, not just displacing them and making demands on their time and their parents' time.

Karen is particularly sensitive to the stress her mother experiences in the caregiving role. In a shared household of this type opportunities for greater stress may exist, but by the same token opportunities for sharing responsibility are also present. There is less conflict in the granddaughter–grandmother relationship than in the daughter–mother relationship, and this can ease the family burden over time.

This balancing of relationships is viewed by Karen from a daughter/ granddaughter stance. As granddaughter, Karen can encourage and persuade her grandmother into desired behavior when her mother, Sarah, is unable to do so. A working through of these "new" relationships is unsettling but productive; as in this story, others can be afforded increased insight and a three dimensional view of those who are carving out new forms of interaction. The mother's/ grandmother's movement toward newly devised forms of interaction does not occur within a vacuum, and Karen notes how it alters the nature of her own interaction within the family.

As Karen moves through the stages of anger and frustration to compromise, understanding, and adjustment she becomes free to accept the exchanges that her grandmother can offer in sharing roots, coping techniques, and love.

Another form of adjustment takes place as this family reaches out to utilize relevant services and resources in the community. The extent and nature of public resources for the elderly and their families will vary from community to community, and though local information may be available regarding the specific services, researching and locating the right help becomes another task for the caregiving family. Sarah and Karen speak of the Adult Day Care Center and its activities, in which Sarah's mother participates, and of the support and information group that they have joined.

Read side by side, Sarah's and Karen's stories are a description not only of their love for Sarah's mother but also of their own caring for each other. As granddaughter, Karen is not the prime caregiver, but she provides both practical assistance as well as understanding and emotional support, as do the other members of the family.

THE BENEFITS OF PROVIDING CARE

The love and concern a family feels for its members is often the motivating force for care of a frail older person.[7] Sarah speaks of the pride and satisfaction she receives from being the caregiver to her mother. A sense of satisfaction in one's actions can lighten the stress that is felt.

Beyond the immediate advantage of accomplishing the goal of providing care, there are other indirect outcomes. Care of an older person nearly always requires involvement of all family members within a household unit and can lead to increased communication and understanding between them. Being a family member in this situation offers a deeper understanding of interpersonal relationships and a sensitivity toward others that will carry over into other situations, under other circumstances, and at other times.

An immediate and obvious benefit to those who hitherto have had no experience of an elderly person is the knowledge of aging that the situation brings. Increased awareness of the needs of elderly persons and a better understanding of what is in store helps the caring family face the future. Karen notes how aware she has become of preventive health care, the universal needs of older people, and the need for families to learn to communicate across generations.

Closely linked to this is the increased awareness of life as a finite passage of time. Facing the image of one's own death may help to conquer and remove death's fear, freeing the self and providing an increased sense of life. Caring for an elderly, frail person provides images and prompts thoughts that may facilitate this process.

Members of a family are interdependent and interact within a unit. In turn, families are interdependent with the outside community. Caring for an older parent can help to bring into focus this wider community. Sarah and Karen discovered a group of supportive friends that connects Sarah and her family with the wider community and underscores the universality of life experiences. The recognition of this is, in itself, a peculiarly healing and sustaining realization. The mother, Sarah, the daughter, Karen, and the other members of the family can only be enriched by this wider support system and the identification with a caregiver constituency.[8]

What is right for one family is not necessarily right for others, however, and while applauding Sarah and her family in their care of Sarah's mother, this is not to find fault with others who opt not to open their homes to an elderly parent.

We need to take a holistic view of the environment of the family, its actual concrete and emotional assets as well as what the priorities are for the total family. Sometimes such a review may not always allow the needs of the older person to come first. What is a plan of choice for one family may differ greatly for another family with the same disabilities and/or assets. Also, priorities for any family may change over time, calling for a new set of plans for the care of the older person.

Past family histories, present responsibilities, family dyanmics and size or practical living arrangements, absence of supportive community services may all dictate against taking an elderly parent into one's home. Other options, such as a nursing home, a retired person's community, a paid companion, or homecare, may offer wiser solutions. In making an informed decision, the wishes and rights of all must be considered—the older person, the prime caregiver, and the other involved family members. The decision as to when and how to provide care to a frail parent is extremely personal.

Whatever the decision, families have identified that the greatest stress is created by the need for emotional support on the part of their older relatives, and that this is the hardest to give. How do the needs of the generations and of the family as a whole mesh with the needs of the disabled older member? Is there conflict or mutual reinforcement? What modifications are required in both physical and emotional environments to meet overall needs?[9] Programs for caregivers, both services on an individual basis and through support groups, demonstrate the need for education and skills training, homecare and respite, and mutual-aid/self-help that can provide emotional support.

With greater longevity we will see more instances of multi-generation families—three- and four-generation families will no longer be rare. Those of us in the service field need to keep in mind the stress levels of each generation's own transitional tasks, identify these stresses, and fashion services that support families through what may be a very difficult period.

REFERENCES

1. Stanley, Cath, "Some Dynamics of the Middle and Later Years," in *Crisis Intervention,* ed. H. J. Parad, (New York: Family Service Association of America, 1965).
2. Sonya L. Rhodes, "A Developmental Approach to the Life Cycle of the Family," *Social Casework* 58, no. 5 (May 1977).
3. Robert Butler and Myrna Lewis, *Aging and Mental Health* (St. Louis. C. V. Mosby, 1977).
4. Elaine Brody, "Women in the Middle and Family Help to Older People," *The Gerontologist* 21, no. 5 (1981):471–80.
5. Amy Horowitz and Rose Dobrof, *Role of Families in Providing Long-Term Care to the Frail and Chronically Ill Elderly Living in the Community.* Final Report to the Health Care Financing Administration, N.Y. Brookdale Center on Aging of Hunter College, 1982.
6. Margaret Blenkner, "Social Work and Family Relationships in Later Life with Some Thoughts on Filial Maturity," in *Social Structure and the Family: Generational Relationships,* ed. G. F. Streib and E. Shanas (Englewood Cliffs, NJ. Prentice Hall, 1965).
7. Elaine Brody, P. T. Johnson, and M. C. Fulcomer, "What Should Adult Children do for Elderly Parents? Opinions and Preferences of Three Generations of Women," *Journal of Gerontology* 39, no. 6 (Nov. 1984).
8. Louis Lowy, "The Older Generation: What is Due, What is Owed," *Social Casework* 64, no. 6 (June 1983).
9. Marjorie Cantor, "Factors Associated with Strain among Family, Friends, and Neighbors Caring for the Frail Elderly." Paper presented at the 34th Annual Scientific Meeting, Gerontological Society, Toronto, 1981.

RECOMMENDED READINGS

Caring: A Family Guide to Managing the Alzheimer's Patient at Home. New York: New York City Department for the Aging, 1985.

Community Service Society, Natural Supports Program. *Caregivers Make the Difference. Group Services for Those Caring for Older Persons in the Community.* Final Report to the Administration on Aging. New York: Community Service Society, 1981.

Strengthening Informal Supports for the Aging. Theory, Practice and Policy Implications. New York: Community Service Society, 1981.

Flint, Margaret M. *A Consumer's Guide to Nursing Home Care in New York City.* Friends and Relatives of the Institutionalized Aged, Inc., 425 East 25th St., New York, NY 10010.

Getzel, George. "Casework with Family Caregivers to the Aged," *Social Casework* 62, no. 4 (April 1981).

Gross-Andrew, Suzannah, and Anna H. Zimmer. "Incentives to Families Caring for Disabled Elderly: Research and Demonstration Project to Strengthen the Natural Support System," *Journal of Gerontological Social Work* 1, no. 2 (Winter 1979).

Hooyman, Nancy, and W. Lustbader. *Taking Care: Supporting Older People and Their Families.* New York: Free Press, 1986.

Horowitz, Amy, and L. Shindelman. "Impact of Caring for an Elderly Relative." Paper presented at the 33rd Annual Scientific meeting, Gerontological Society, San Diego, 1980.

Mellor, Joanna, and George Getzel. "Stress and Service Needs of Those Who Care for the Aged." Paper presented at the 33rd Annual Scientific meeting, Gerontological Society, San Diego, 1980.

Mellor, M. Joanna, Harriet Rzetelny, and Iris Hudis. "Self-Help Groups for Caregivers of the Aged" in *The Self-Help Revolution,* ed. F. Riessman and A. Gartner. New York: Human Sciences Press, 1984.

Silverstone, B., and H. Hyman. *You and Your Aging Parent.* Rev. and enl. ed. New York: Pantheon, 1982.

RESOURCES

New York City Department for the Aging:
 Information and Referral—(212) 577-0800
 Alzheimer's Resource Center—(212) 577-7564
New York City Self-Help Clearing House, 186 Joralemon St., Brooklyn, NY 12201. (718) 852-4290.
New York State Office for the Aging
 Senior Citizen Hotline: 1-800-342-9871

It Was a Wild
and Woolly Country

Carrie

Carrie, Sarah's mother, spent an evening talking with the daughters' group. She reminisced about early times—a move to Oklahoma in 1905 with scary memories and a tragic ending in the loss of both her sisters to typhoid and then the return to Indiana. She tells the story of her young adulthood, of caring for her own parents and her children, and of the recent illness and death of her husband. And she talks about what it is like for her now in her new home with her own belongings—her quilts and furniture—"a nice big looking-glass . . . and my old rocking chair . . . and my bed . . . it's a good bed. I've got all those things in my bedroom."

Carrie was pleased to know that her story would be told with Sarah's and Karen's. The following is an adaptation of the taped conversation of that evening. Questions from the group are included.

THE EARLY YEARS

Daughter: Tell us about your parents, Carrie.
Carrie: Both of my parents came from Germany. Pa was a cabinet maker and he learned that trade in school. He had a tragic accident and had all the fingers cut off his left hand. He was not able to use all the machinery in the furniture factory where he worked . . . so he did mostly repair work in the factory. Mom and Dad were good savers, and they owned their own little farm in Indiana close to the town where I was born. I was the youngest of four children. Mom was close to forty when I was born, and my brother and two sisters were quite a bit older than me. My older sister, Stella, was married and had her divorce. . . . She was living

25

at home with her new baby . . . Virginia was born at our house. . . . My niece and I were like sisters because Mom raised her after Stella died.

We'd take my dad to work in the factory every day, and that's the way we got along. And we had a nice home. We had a good living. But Dad wanted my brother with rheumatism to live in a warmer climate, and my sister had to get away to start a new life . . . so we moved to Oklahoma. I was seven.

Daughter: Did you ride the train out there from here?

Carrie: Yes. Dad had a box car rented on the train and . . . let's see, did we have a team of horses? I think we had a team. . . . No, no, I take it back. We had just the one horse, and I think we had two cows. We went down there and went to a little town. It was ten miles away from the land Dad bought. My dad rented a house for us to stay in while he and my brother built a house on his land. He bought two teams of horses, one for himself and one for my brother.

Daughter: What was the town like?

Carrie: There was just a little trail there in town . . . a grocery store and a house or two. It wasn't a regular town. You couldn't buy any dry goods or anything like that there. It was just a little burg.

Daughter: Where did you go to buy your dry goods and things like that?

Carrie: Once or twice a year we went to a bigger town. There was a general store and a post office. . . . No, not a post office . . . a train depot. . . . We had to walk to school. Down there where we lived there were just trails. . . .

Daughter: Did you have a pony?

Carrie: No, I didn't have a pony then. I had one at last, but I didn't have one then . . . I had to walk. We had to walk—with the wolves . . . and the coyotes . . . and things like that, you know. And the cattle—the cattle were the worst thing. The cattle would run the wolves off or take after them. But then, I was afraid of the cattle too. We would go along the fence row, the barbed wire fence we had down there. I had to go along through the fence row, you know, to keep away—hide . . . well, not hide, but get away from them chasing me.

Daughter: Did you help your mother? Did you have a lot of chores to do?

Carrie: I was just a kid, you know, to begin with, but then, *my land yes! We all had to work*—Dad needed us. My dad, he just had one hand, but you know he could handle himself pretty good—with his other hand.

Daughter: Did you get a lot of rain?

Carrie: It was dry country. And when we got rain one year, we was just washed out. Course Dad had nothing but failing crops.

Daughter: Did you have a lot of trouble with grasshoppers?

Carrie: We had trouble with *all insects*. We lived on ducks and geese. . . . Dad built a pond close to the house. They had to build our house on the side of a hill, and a little ways away, he dug a pond. We practically lived on them (ducks and geese) in the winter time. My dad would only kill two hogs a year for the whole family because we had so much wildlife.

Daughter: He sold the hogs?

Carrie: Yes, he would sell everything he could to make a living.

Daughter: He was a homesteader, wasn't he?

Carrie: Yes, he had one hundred acres and . . . there was a lot to do. He dug rocks so much of the time—to clear land so he could plant more.

Daughter: Were there any trees out there at all?

Carrie: None. No trees. There weren't very many trees anywhere.

Daughter: Did you have a well for water?

Carrie: Yes, he dug a well . . . course, in the summertime we always hauled our water. We had to go a couple of miles to haul the water. It was from a spring, you might say. It supplied practically the whole neighborhood, but not many people lived around there. Mom used to catch rain water sometimes to wash with—*if* it rained! The livestock died down there as fast as you could buy them, that is, cows and horses, 'cause they was . . . you know they had fevers and things like that out on the prairie. That was rough country!!!

Daughter: That made a hard transition for you, didn't it?

Carrie: That's right. I was scared to go past them rock piles my dad had.

Daughter: Were there snakes?

Carrie: Snakes! We learned how to run from them. Yes, there were snakes, skunks, too.

Daughter: And rabbits. Did you eat rabbits?

Carrie: Yes, the rabbits wasn't as good as the ducks. We about lived on ducks and wild geese. . . . I can just see Dad creeping down to the pond yet. . . . He always killed several ducks if they didn't get away before he got there. . . . It was fun for him but, oh, how sick we girls used to get cleaning ducks and rabbits.

Daughter: Would the jack rabbits eat your grain?

Carrie: Oh yes, yes. That's what we had dogs for. The dogs would run them off.

Daughter: Did you ever have your own hens and chickens out in Oklahoma?

Carrie: Yes, uh-huh. We had . . . Mom had to raise them. We never had them to sell though. The coyotes and wolves would get too many. We could never raise enough.

Daughter: Hawks, too, I'll bet.

Carrie: Hawks, yes, but it was the wolves who would come at night.

Daughter: Your mother had a wonderful garden and orchard in Indiana. What was it like for her when she went to Oklahoma then? Was she able to have a garden in Oklahoma?

Carrie: Yes, yes. . . . She gardened. . . . She always had a garden out there. And we picked berries—it was fun to pick berries.

Daughter: Did she ever say she was discouraged or anything?

Carrie: Oh, yes, we were all a little bit discouraged, but we didn't dare say it around Dad because he was doing the best he could.

Daughter: A lot of bad things happened to you down there, didn't they?

Carrie: I had two sisters that died just a few weeks apart. They had typhoid fever. . . . One died the fifth of July [1911] and the other along about the

fifteenth of August. . . . We all had typhoid fever, and there was nothing the doctors could do about it. We just had to wear it out, and I was pretty bad . . . when my second sister died, why I was sick. I couldn't go to her funeral. . . . And I didn't get any better till, oh, along about October or November. I couldn't walk and I was helpless. . . . I didn't have any memory or anything . . . they didn't think I would live. My daddy used to have to carry me around till I got well enough to walk. And I was a big girl. And Mom would put me in the wheelbarrow and push me down to the garden. . . . And Virginia, my niece . . . Mom had Virginia to raise and Virginia had typhoid fever, too. Then, oh, about Christmas time they got me to walking. I didn't get to go to school that year, and I couldn't go back to school the first of the year. I was just an invalid for awhile. My legs . . . I didn't have good use of my legs 'cause there wasn't any strength in my legs. I had passed the sixth grade when I had typhoid fever. And the year before my two sisters, my niece, and I all had scarlet fever.
Daughter: Did you want to come back to Indiana?
Carrie: Didn't have any choice. We came back because we just got to the place where my daddy said soon after my sisters died, why—we've got to go back to Indiana—I shouldn't say anything about that. [She cries.] It makes me feel bad to talk about it. My sisters—we brought one of them back—brought her body back. And the other one, my brother brought her back.

Carrie's brother John had returned from Oklahoma to Indiana and found a job. His rheumatic problem had responded well to the southwestern climate, but John had grown restless there. As Carrie said, "He didn't like the country down there and he came back [to Indiana] because he liked to play ball and things like that . . . and he went back to the factory . . . and got his old friends back . . . and girls."

In June 1911, John married one of the girls, Tillie, and took his young bride to Oklahoma to meet his family. On arrival, they discovered they would not be permitted to enter his parents' home because of the typhoid fever. Stella died while they were in the area, and it became the unhappy duty of the newlyweds to convey her body back to Indiana for burial.

Although life in the Southwest was very hard, Carrie has memories of good times as well. She recalls parties where the young people would dance, and visits with neighbors on the way to and from school were also special. Eventually, there was a pony, Billy, and when Billy had to be sold on the return to Indiana, "It like to broke my heart," Carrie says now.

Carrie and her family moved back to Indiana in 1912 to discover that John's "rheumatism" had flared up again, and he was unable to work. Baby Frank had arrived, and Tillie was forced to find a job. Carrie was not permitted to return to school, but was left at home to take care of the baby while all of the other family members sought employment.

BACK IN INDIANA

Carrie: Mom had to go to work. . . . John and Tillie had a baby and I had that youngster to take care of. . . . I was just a kid myself and I practically raised Frank. . . . I should have been in school but Mom needed me at home.
Mom was a nurse and had to help Dad get back on his feet. We had hard times. . . . Mom went out nursing and left me with Frank and Virginia—course *she* went to school. . . . And Dad, he worked in the factory, and I kept his meals up for him and fixed him his lunch to take.
Daughter: So it was really hard for you not to be able to go to school.
Carrie: *I didn't have a chance.* I didn't have any trouble going to school but I couldn't get to school 'cause the kids had to be taken care of. . . . We had hard times. . . . I took care of Frank, and I was so sick and tired of taking care of that kid. . . . I was sick and tired of taking care of Virginia too.

Eventually John became a bedfast invalid, Tillie departed with young Frank, and Carrie's mother decided to stay home and nurse John. Carrie (now seventeen) seized the opportunity to get out of the house, going to work first in a glove factory and later in a cigar factory where the pay was better. She is still enthusiastic about her work experience: "I could make gloves in my sleep."

Carrie: Well, they think because you work in a cigar factory that you like tobacco. But you can't—you can't even get a taste of it, or it makes you sick to your stomach. When you get the bunches, they put the cigars in trays . . . and you get twelve in a bunch or a tray, and you get so much a tray for wrapping them. Why, I just loved making cigars!

Carrie recalls the financial rewards with relish. By the time she married Leonard in 1926 after a seven-year courtship, Carrie had bought and paid for a four-room house and a Model T Ford.

Daughter: You earned enough money at the factory to buy a car, didn't you?
Carrie: I bought more than a car. I bought my home. I bought my home.
Daughter: So you started out your married life in your own home.
Carrie: I spent my money on that house, and I paid for it. . . . I can't remember just all that I did to it. I know I papered that house and put fencing around it. . . . I just did things. . . . We lived there and had our children there. And my husband worked hard. He was a countryman's boy. Leonard always worked someplace. . . . He drove a truck, a gasoline truck out through the country, and we made a good living. And I worked! I had two children, but then I didn't neglect them. I stayed home and raised them till they were old enough to go to school.
Daughter: You took a few years off and raised the children. That would be Sarah and Linda. Was Sarah the elder?

Carrie: Sarah's the youngest. My oldest girl died. She died about eights months before Leonard did. Oh, so much happened during that time I can't. . . . [weeps]

Before her marriage to Leonard, Carrie's father had to leave his factory job. Her parents then moved out to the country.

Carrie: I would go out there every week—ten miles out—they just had a little ten-acre place. . . . They were living on a shoestring, and I would go out and take them groceries and such. I drove, and I had a Ford car that I bought new, and I wore it out [laughter]. And Leonard—I had an awful good husband. He didn't make a whole lot of money, but we had a good living. And we just helped them out the best we could. And they of course had a horse and buggy and could go to the store. And they had their neighbors to bring in groceries.
Daughter: And then you had your own children. . . .
Carrie: Yes, when my two children were born, Mom would fix Dad a lot to eat to run him for awhile, and then she'd come down and help me out. Leonard would go out and get her and she'd help me awhile. That's the way we'd manage. We always was a family that took care of ourselves. We never depended on anybody else, only ourselves.
Daughter: So your mother helped to deliver your babies.
Carrie: Yes, she did. Dad would just "batch it" and she'd come into town and help me over the worst of it. Then she'd pull out, and I kind of had to help myself. . . . Of course, I helped them out when they were in trouble.
Daughter: What happened with your parents? How did you know that they couldn't stay by themselves any more?
Carrie: Well, I would go out there every week. . . . But Mother and Dad both got down—they were old when they died. . . . I never had to support my folks, but I took care of them when they were sick, and took them into my home. . . . I took care of them till they died.

Carrie's father died at the age of eighty-one in 1936. Her mother, who apparently was able to do household chores such as babysitting, died two years later at the age of seventy-seven. Carrie was able to sell the country property, and this sale helped her to acquire a larger home for her family. There she lived in a close neighborhood setting until her husband's illness.

As Sarah points out, Carrie's family-centered, small-town existence came to an end in the early 1980s. Daughter Linda lost her battle with cancer while Leonard developed Parkinson's Disease. Carrie endeavored to care for her husband: "I had an awful time with him. I had an awful time getting him out of bed, the urinal, chairs. . . ." However, after developing serious hypertension and other illnesses herself, she had to give up the struggle, and Leonard was placed in a nursing home. Carrie went to live with Sarah and her family in the suburbs of a small city.

Carrie has found some difficulties in adjusting to her new lifestyle. As she tells it, the unfamiliar technology of her daughter's home is responsible, but clearly she is aware that she has suffered some impairments.

A NEW LIFESTYLE

Daughter: So you are staying with Sarah, as your mother stayed with you, and helping.

Carrie: I'm not helping now. I can't . . . that stove is driving me nuts. I can't get used to that stove. If they had a gas stove, it would be different.

Daughter: Do you like to cook? Do you miss cooking?

Carrie: I like to cook but I've forgotten how. . . . Well, I tell you, I wasn't in very good health when Sarah brought me down here—when I first was here—but she's taken me to the doctor, and he's done a lot for me. Straightened my mind out a little bit for me. So I know more about what I'm doin' than what I did before.

Daughter: Well, you've had some really hard times. You went through all that with your husband, and then you had an infection.

Carrie: That's right. That's right.

Daughter: That can do bad things to us.

Carrie: Yes, I'm just so now that I can help with the dishes, but they have a dishwasher. . . . They just pick up the dishes and stick them in the dishwasher, you know. . . . I could wash dishes like we washed dishes at home.

Carrie explained that "Sarah's been awful good to me. Sarah and Jim both and the children are good to me. . . . She's given me the best room in the house."

Carrie went on to say that "the stairs are kind of hard sometimes," as is the moderately steep hill outside the suburban home. She reminisced about her own home which had to be sold when she moved, and then conceded that she couldn't care for herself there now.

Daughter: Well, Carrie, I know you are getting tired. I'll call Sarah and tell her that we are just about talked out. I want to tell you, though, that we appreciate your coming to talk with us. . . . We don't often get a chance to talk with someone who has seen the things you have seen and lived the way you have lived.

Carrie: That's right. It was a wild and woolly country.

The Importance of
Reminiscence and
Family Tradition

Dixie Kline Richardson

A mind that seems to be dwelling on the past is no longer thought of as an idiosyncrasy of advancing age or "senile" behavior, but as a normal, natural, and healthy occupation as human beings contemplate the end of their life span. This reviewing of one's life—Paul Tournier in *The Meaning of Persons* speaks of the "recounting of a lifestory"[1]—is a process in which we attempt to summarize our lives in search of purpose and meaning. According to Myrna I. Lewis and Robert N. Butler, "there is a consensus that older persons are psychologically fragile. However, we often fail to remember that older persons are master survivors compared to the young. Older people have the capacity to reconcile their lives, to confront real guilt and find meaning, especially in the presence of acceptance and support from others." They point out also that "there is a real sense of putting one's life in order through this [life] review."[2]

My maternal grandmother was dying of cancer in 1964. Because it had metastasized into her spine, her last days were spent in severe pain. My time with her was precious. At age twenty-five I was about to lose one of the people in my life who had been a strong role model. I had five living grandparents when my first child was born, but this woman and I were extremely close. I was her first

Dixie Kline Richardson has been a journalist, genealogist, historian, collector of folklore, bereavement counselor, older adult specialist, mental health consultant, and educator. She is the wife of a school teacher, the mother of two sons and a daughter, and the grandmother of four children.

grandchild. "Tell me about the time. . . ." I asked her again for a story from her childhood. The grimace of pain eased from her face, she settled back, folded her hands against her chest, and I watched reminiscing act as a tranquilizer while she revisited happy, golden years. Twenty-three years later, I still find my speech peppered with stories, witticisms, and expressions that were uniquely hers; and I miss her. As I experience my own aging and grandmotherhood, I appreciate more and more the rich and varied legacy of values and lore, the traditions that she and others passed to me; and I realize my good fortune in having been reared in a family with available and accessible parents, grandparents, and uncles and aunts of several generations. They recounted their lives and the lives of others I never knew—lives whose characters and events influenced mine. From this heritage, I have known who I am.

We are all shaped by the past. That which affected our ancestors has had direct consequences in our lives. There are more things handed down than red hair and streaks of stubbornness, or Haviland china and Uncle Harvey's gold watch. These patterns of influence have come from significant and life-changing events, family belief systems and rituals, ethnic origins, places of residence, socio-economic situations, and personal decisions made by those who came before us. Being a link between the past and future, each of us must bear in mind that every time someone dies (or suffers total devastation of the faculty of memory), a lifetime of facts, experience, and memories from a particular historical and cultural period is lost forever. Each of us has a life story no one else can tell. Separation and death may also take from us, or change, some of the family rituals, traditions, and celebrations that hold us together and identify us as a family. Alex Shoumatoff in *The Mountain of Names: A History of the Human Family*,[3] writes of the warmth, support, and stability that "intact" families give their members. Anthropologist Margaret Mead wrote that a student poignantly reported, "My grandmother planted my roots in the earth." This basic need for being grounded is graphic in the suicide note left by a youngster who hanged himself from a tree: "This is the only thing around here with roots."

I see reminiscing as being a testimony to human potential and a celebration of life's personal meaning. I believe valuing and carrying on special family traditions and rituals reinforces our individual and familial sense of identity and security. For the institutionalized person, a loss perhaps overlooked by the family is that he or she may be left out of family celebrations. Or consider another deprivation—that of having no one left who knew you when you were young.

Among our basic needs is that desire to be appreciated and accepted as we are and for all we have been; the effort to keep intact one's unique personality extends throughout life. To review the broad spectrum of our entirety—who we are, including our deficits as well as strengths—we require witnesses, those who are interested and supportive listeners. Reminiscing gives us the means of seeing an older adult as he or she once was (those self-images stay with us). It is a means of preserving and perpetuating heritage and tradition because, as the oldest or last link in the family's chain to the past, the elderly person is a living archive. The senior members of the family carry not only their memories, but the inherited memories of those long gone. Reminiscing can bring youth and age together in a bond that validates both generations. (Have you observed that unconditional love which so often exists between grandparent and grand-child?)

Dispelling the loneliness of unshared memories, reminiscing can be a socialization tool. It can aid orientation, in that a good grip on the past may help in adapting to the stresses and changes of the present. One's sense of self-worth and personal integrity are buttressed when accomplishments are realized and recognized, when human frailties and weaknesses are accepted without judgment or condemnation, and when opinions are heard and valued. As a coping mechanism, reviewing one's life can help resolve, or at least release, the pain of old conflicts, leftover disappointments and loss and can be a vital part of getting one's "final affairs" in order. This may be uncomfortable or painful for the listener, but being heard in a nonjudgmental, caring, and supportive atmosphere may be that older person's last opportunity to die at peace with self and others. This is a gift you can give; learn to be comfortable with your discomfort! In these instances we need to know that it is not our advice and counsel that are sought so much as warmth, empathy, and a willingness to hear. Being gentle in this kind of "witnessing" situation, we may not have to remind ourselves that our time will also come. This recounting can be an affirmation of rich significance for those who recall and share the struggles and fears of both failure and success over a lifetime and can be life-affirming to those who listen. Rest assured you will gain insight into "survivorship." A caveat—if your elderly relative seems stuck or is excessively wrestling with some area of the past, this may be a signal for some professional assessment and counseling to address the need for resolution.

The stories we are told can depict the character of individual family members and the family as a whole. Life review will describe the pivotal points that chart the course (the events that are life's milestones) and the everyday trivia of human existence that are experienced universally. We are often delighted to learn the origins of some of the particular rituals we take for granted. We may be surprised to discover how some members fell into, chose, or were delegated to the roles they play within the family. The revelation of turning points, personalities, traditions, and everyday trivia unique to our families certifies for us a sense of continuity, connectedness, and belonging. These feelings are basic to our whole-ness and will be a by-product for the persons reminiscing as well as for those who share it. It must be stressed that even the mentally impaired will frequently have clear, lucid, and vivid recall, and being able to talk with someone who wants to hear them boosts their self-esteem, makes them feel valued and less isolated. They, especially, need to experience the security of feeling anchored. I think here of the saddest statement I hear from those elderly people, sound or impaired, who tell me, "I am the last of my family."

"I do not live in the past; it is the past which is alive in me," said René Dubos.[4] As the end of life approaches, or as we come to the sudden realization that our older relatives are not always going to be with us, it is a common occurrence that we begin to think of family history. How many times I have heard these words spoken: "I wish . . . that I had asked . . . that I had listened . . . that I had written it down." As you begin to collect history or want to encourage reminiscing, topics that can be an impetus (and which you should think about in documenting your own story) are practice, tradition, experience, belief, and ritual in regard to parent-child relationships, youthful passages, courtship and marriage (do you know how your parents met?), the Depression and war years (indeed life-changing events), holidays, entertainment, education, religion, professions, and death and dying (this is the chance to ask about life-support system decisions). Ask your relative (and yourself), "What do you want to be remembered for?" Another caveat—never trust your memory; get this down on paper and keep duplicates. Tape records are helpful; videotapes are a priceless visual memento. To make this pursuit easier, cleverly designed bound volumes are a wonderful record and keepsake. These can be found in bookstores or obtained from genealogical publishers. With the extension of life today, it is not too far-fetched a possibility that children can know and interact with their eight great-grandparents. Generally, a great many people do not even know the names of those eight whose joining created them.

We live in an era of rapid change, displaced and disrupted family ties, shifting values and expectations, rootlessness and uncertainty, and we all face the possibility of losing those who knew us when we were young. Death, divorce, relocation, children leaving the nest can precipitate the giving up of treasured traditions, celebrations, close and potentially enriching relationships. These vacuums need to be filled. Families break apart; new families are created. New ways of celebrating and continuing tradition, of feeling connected and grounded are necessary. (A friend is adamant in her advice to engaged couples. Never marry, she says, until it's decided how to spend Christmas with both sets of parents.)

To help ourselves and to help escort the old and our young through life's stages and transitions, it is important to: hear and share the testimony of survivorship, feel part of a continuum, create and maintain traditions that reinforce the strength of family, and to have the certitude and dignity that come from being cherished as the unique and precious persons that we are.

REFERENCES

1. Paul Tournier, *The Meaning of Persons* (New York: Harper & Brothers, 1957.
2. Myrna I. Lewis, and Robert N. Butler, "Life Review Therapy: Putting Memory to Work in Individual and Group Psychotherapy." *Geriatrics* 29, No. 11 (1974): 199–205.
3. Alex Shoumatoff, *The Mountain of Names: A History of the Human Family,* (New York: Simon & Schuster, 1986).
4. René Dubos, *Celebrations of Life* (New York: McGraw-Hill, 1981).

RECOMMENDED READINGS

Blythe, Ronald. *View in Winter*. New York: Harcourt Brace Jovanovich, 1979.
Howard, Jane. *Families*. New York: Simon and Schuster, 1978.
Kaminsky, Mark, ed. *The Uses of Reminiscence: New Ways of Working with Older Adults*. New York: Haworth Press, 1984.
Talbot, Toby. *A Book about My Mother*. New York: Farrar, Straus and Giroux, 1980.
Viorst, Judith. *Necessary Losses*. New York: Simon and Schuster, 1986.

Issues in Health and Illness
Ellen Beck

I, too, am a daughter of the elderly. I was born when my mother was forty-three and my father fifty-three. Thus, I started to learn about aging as I was growing up. When I was a resident in family medicine, I was asked to give a series of lectures in health to a group of elderly people at our local Golden Age Association. I learned so much from them. They were avid, open, eager learners.

Is it possible to achieve well-being, to achieve joy, to face the obstacles that aging presents?

Health, according to the WHO (World Health Organization), is not simply the absence of disease but, rather, the presence of a state of well-being. Thus, health can be seen as having physical, psychological, spiritual, and social components.

When we think of aging, we must think of it as a time in which each of these aspects of health may be threatened but also in which each of these aspects has a capacity for growth. Aging involves the loss of physical capacity and reserve and the possibility of overcoming and adapting to these losses. It involves the loss of numerous sources of self-esteem, of roles, and the loss of a social support network and the potential for evolution at a spiritual level.

When you ask people of any age, "Do you feel old?" they usually will say "No." If you ask them, "What would happen to make you feel old?" often they will say, "Loss of function, loss of independence, loss of physical health." In fact, I think we often equate the word "old" with "sick." How many of us on a cold, dreary morning will wake up with an aching back and head and say, "Oh, do I feel old today."

Ellen Beck, MD, family physician and teacher, is an assistant professor in the Department of Family Medicine, McGill University. She is a daughter of elderly parents, a wife, and mother of two babies. She loves to dance, talk, write, and sit on cliffs overlooking the ocean. She sees herself as a learner and occasional teacher on the wonderful journey that is life.

What is the reality? There is a reality associated with aging—a physical reality of loss of certain functions, changes in others, and increasing susceptibility to, or chance of, certain illnesses. Many older people, when asked their greatest fear, do not say death but rather illness, incapacity, dependence, the loss of capacity to function independently. These are the true diseases of old age, the inability to walk as one would like, to do as much as one would like, to be limited by fear, pain, and weakness.

There is also the concept of illness versus disease. Disease is the actual pathological (physical) diagnosis, for example, liver disease or kidney disease. Illness is the subjective feeling of an absence of well-being characterized by the sentence, "I don't feel well." So often, we go to a physician not feeling well. Cancer or some terrible disease is ruled out. Nonetheless, we still leave the office feeling ill.

Our sense of illness may be because of psychological, physical, or spiritual pain. But somehow, these other aspects often do not enter in the medical domain; often the response may be a tranquilizer or a painkiller (treating the symptoms instead of helping you explore the cause).

Given the importance of the individual sense of independence and the individual subjective feelings of illness that people experience, it is important that each of us become enablers in our lives. First, we must identify what health means for each of us and then do our utmost to achieve it. To be enablers is to create an environment in which the individuals can take maximum responsibility themselves. Then we can go on to become enablers at other levels of responsibility: family, culture, community, and society.

One other comment: medicine is a field of the unknown. Physicians and scientists are trying to unravel an unknowable mystery, the human body, and the more we find out, the more we realize the nascent level of our understanding. This perspective means that much of what I am going to explain in this chapter is a way of understanding a problem. But in no way is it "truth." Moreover, so often when we go to the physician we go wanting a concrete answer to a problem, and the physician wants to be able to give a concrete answer. The patient finds it hard to hear, "I don't know," and the physician finds it just as hard to say it.

NORMAL AGING

People often ask me: "What's normal aging? How do you distinguish normal from abnormal?" When they ask this question, it seems to me that they are not asking, "How does the liver change with aging?" or "How many skin cells die each year?" but rather "If I or someone I love has a symptom or something seems wrong, how do I know whether I should go to the doctor and have it checked out, how do I know if it's something to worry about?"

Well, there are a few basic rules to follow:

1) Aging, in general, is a time of decreased flexibility, decreased rapidity of response, and decreased reserve capacity to overcome prolonged stress. However, unless you have a particular problem or disease, everything still works. It just works a little more slowly, takes a little longer to get going, and does not have as much staying power. These principles are just as true for waking up in the morning as they are for our sex lives. Our physical organs respond in the same way.

2) Nonetheless, if you have a symptom that decreases your functioning or worries you, go see a physician, preferably a family physician or a geriatrician (who specializes in the care of older adults), and check it out. The question "What do you expect at your age?" should be thrown into the garbage can. If someone says to you "What do you expect at your age?" the response is: "I expect to feel good as long as I can. I know I have limitations but when something new goes wrong, I want to know if it can be fixed or what I can do to help deal with it."

3) Therefore, all new symptoms should be checked out. Don't feel embarrassed or intimidated. Sometimes the physician's seeming disinterest stems from a frustration at not knowing exactly what is going on or at being unable to help. You may ask, "Why go to the trouble of checking it out?" The reason is that for each symptom, there are always some irreversible causes and some *reversible* ones. This is true for hearing loss, dementia, memory loss, impotence, urinary incontinence (loss), constipation, chest pain, and so on. The list is endless. It is the possibility of a reversible cause that makes it *always* worthwhile to check out the symptom. If nothing can be done, so be it. But check it out first.

In aging, we must deal with many losses. I have felt for a long time that the loss that is relatively unique to aging is the loss of one's physical capacity. Although throughout one's life one has to deal with loss, these losses are external—losses in one's milieu, but not losses in the inner sanctuary of the body. But with aging come losses within oneself. So even though many of us say, "As long as I have my health, I can cope with anything," with true physiological aging comes the loss of one's physical capacity and autonomy.

To maintain a sense of well-being, a sense of "health" despite all this is not an easy task. It is nonetheless possible and, if we are ready to take on the challenge, attainable.

Eventually, as aging progresses, we address the ultimate loss of our life— death, the loss of one's physical existence; aging is the preparation for this loss. To still achieve health, a state and sense of well-being in the sanctuary that is our body at this stage of life is not easy. It requires doing whatever prevention we can, acknowledging the limitations of our body, taking care of ourselves in a way that has never been necessary before, and finding meaning and beauty in our lives, a beauty tinged with—and perhaps more beautiful because of—our imminent sense of our own mortality.

MEDICATION

Many older people are over-medicated, either by themselves or by their physicians. Why is this? There are several reasons: With aging, the body is less able to handle drugs. The kidneys and the liver are the body's clearing houses. With aging, their capacity to "throw out the garbage" slows down. Thus, a person needs less medication (that is lower doses) to have the same effect. Also, it is easier to treat the symptom than explore, discover, and treat its cause. This principle is just the same for patients as it is for physicians. How often when we get a headache, do we simply take an aspirin to make the headache go away instead of saying, "OK, head, what message do you have for me and how should I cope with it?"

Deep down, I think many of us wish for "magic bullets," that is, pills that make the problem go away completely, right away. In reality, very few magic bullets exist (and believe me, physicians wish for them as much as patients). This is especially true in terms of mental illness. If we are feeling anxious or depressed, often the physician's response will be to prescribe a tranquilizer (for anxiety) or an antidepressant. But maybe, what we really need to do is explore the causes of our anxiety or depression. This may require psychotherapy or counseling with an experienced therapist, psychologist, or psychiatrist. But I believe it is always worth the effort. Many people, professionals and elderly alike, respond, "Therapy, what, at my age! You must be crazy." But it has been my consistent experience that if a person is willing to take charge of her/his life, face reality squarely in the face and learn to cope, the results can be wonderful, *at any age*. As long as we are alive and our mind works, we can learn and grow.

To get back to medicines, all drugs have side effects, that is, all drugs (like everything in life) have benefits and drawbacks. You have to weigh the one against the other. An unexplained symptom occurring soon or even quite awhile after starting a new drug is always worth checking out with your physician. The following are some classic examples of often-used drugs and their little-known side effects:

> —Cimetidine (Tagamet), an excellent drug used for treatment of ulcers, can cause confusion, especially in the elderly patient.
> —Valium (Diazepam) used as a tranquilizer for anxiety can unmask a masked depression, that is, can bring out depressive symptoms.
> —Aldomet (Alpha-methyldopa), a drug commonly used for high blood pressure, can cause depression and impotence.
> —Aspirin can cause ulcers.

Beware of multiplying drugs: often one drug is given for the side effects of another drug instead of considering stopping the first drug. In this way the person ends up taking several drugs, each one for the side effects of the previous one.

If you are taking a drug, and you think it is causing certain unpleasant side effects, do not stop the drug suddenly on your own. Check with your doctor first. Some drugs have rebound effects, so that when you stop them suddenly your symptoms suddenly get much worse. A classic example of this is Inderal (propanolol) when used for angina (chest pain). These drugs must be tapered slowly, that is, decreased a little at a time before stopping the drug completely.

Physicians often talk about drug compliance. This means whether the patient is actually taking the drug and complying with the "doctor's orders." Many people, although they are not taking the drug exactly as prescribed or perhaps not at all, choose not to tell their physician. Perhaps they feel he or she will be angry or critical. I believe that this behavior doesn't pay off in the long run. If you don't like what you are taking, say so. If not, it can work against you. The physician may raise the dose or try something stronger thinking that the drug is not working.

Remember there are two main categories of medication: drugs that fix things (therapeutic drugs) and drugs that treat symptoms (palliative drugs). The first group tend to be drugs that we need to take to treat a condition, for example, antibiotics for a bacterial infection like pneumonia or a urinary infection, insulin for diabetes, anti-hypertensives for high blood pressure. Although I believe in minimizing medication, it is still worthwhile and important to take this type of medication. The other big group of drugs are for symptoms. These include pain-killers, tranquilizers, and laxatives. With these pills, we have much more of a choice. Medication is one approach but it does not make the problem go away; it just makes it easier to live with. This can be a two-edged sword. The easier a problem is to live with, the less likely you are to explore its roots, the more likely you are to start getting used to the medication, and the more likely you are to continue to expose yourself to whatever is causing the problem thereby making the problem worse and increasing the need for drugs.

Let's review some basic principles.

1) Know what you are taking. This stuff is going into your body; it's up to you to find out about it. Know the name, dose, and why you are taking it. These days, I think people read the labels on the food they buy much more diligently than they learn about what medicines they're taking.

2) If an unpleasant symptom occurs, make sure that it is not a side effect of a medication. The best way to do this (usually) is by checking it out with your doctor.

3) Older people usually need lower doses of drugs than younger people.

4) All drugs have good effects and bad effects. The "perfect drug" does not exist.

5) If your elderly family members can no longer see or remember as well as previously, devise a system using envelopes or colored boxes so that they don't get mixed up with their medication.

6) Many medications cause drowsiness and lethargy, and can contribute to

confusion or mimic dementia. These drugs (all drugs, for that matter) should be minimized in the elderly person.

7) Know the difference between a therapeutic drug and a symptomatic one. Know why you have to take it and decide for yourself (with your physician) whether you truly need it. For example, drugs for high blood pressure are being taken to prevent strokes. This has always seemed to me to be a pretty good reason to take them.

8) Know what you can do to help treat the problem without drugs or at least, to minimize the amount needed (for example, weight loss and low salt diet in terms of high blood pressure; weight loss for diabetes and arthritis).

9) Explore the possible causes of a problem, and see if you can change the situation before you decide to use a medication. This is particularly true for physical symptoms caused primarily by psychological stress. *Listen* to your body; it can be very smart.

10) Once your problem has been diagnosed by a doctor, consider exploring alternative methods of treatment that do not require drugs (for example, biofeedback for high blood pressure, autogenic therapy for migraines or insomnia).

To summarize: (1) minimize medications; (2) the more you know, the better; and (3) never forget, *you* own your body. Make sure that what goes into it is good for it.

AGING AND MENTAL HEALTH

To me, mental health means quite simply a sense of well-being. Whatever the cause, mental illness is a devastating problem and we understand it very poorly.

To be the daughter of someone with a mental health problem is very difficult. You see them in their fear, anxiety, grief, or pain and often feel totally powerless to help them—you want to, you reach out, you try, but somehow it is not heard or is pushed away. Often the road from mental illness to mental health (like life itself) is one we must ultimately travel alone—hopefully we have friends, supporters, and helpers along the way. To see your parent severely depressed or anxious is frightening at many levels:

Could it happen to me?
What's happening to her?
I can't stand seeing him like this.
I'm angry at her for becoming like this.
I'm ashamed to tell people.
Now he's going to be a burden to me. I'll have no freedom.

What can you do to help? First, face your own feelings and reactions. If necessary, perhaps it would be good for you to speak to a therapist, counselor, or social worker—someone with whom you can lay down your burden. Hopefully, facing your feelings will help you forgive and face your parent and truly help her/him.

Sometimes, our only alternative is to wait and hope. Do not be afraid to reach out to him or her in a time of pain and anguish. It is much less lonely to cry together than alone, and don't be afraid they'll become too dependent on you (or you on them). The time will pass, situations will change, and you both will change.

You must be an advocate for your elderly parent in the medical situation. If they are rejecting you or denying your existence, try to forgive them and accept them as they are in whatever relationship they will allow. Here too, patience is of great importance. You must be their advocate, their friend, and at the same time take care of your own needs.

Some general rules relating to mental health problems follow:

1) As always, be an advocate for your parent. Make sure all their medications are checked as possible causes of the problem. Make sure they have appropriate blood tests and so on to rule out physical causes of mental illness symptoms.

2) Do *not* assume they are becoming demented—often symptoms of depression in the elderly mimic dementia.

3) Nonetheless, make sure dementia is ruled out.

4) See someone who cares about the problems of mental illness in the elderly— sometimes "the best psychiatrist in the city" is not necessarily the best person to see your parent. A good book to read on this is *What Happened to My Mother* by Henry Edward (Harper and Row, 1981).

5) If you do not feel intuitively comfortable with the treating physician or psychiatrist, get a second opinion. A clinical psychologist, counselor, social worker, or chaplain can often offer a useful perspective.

6) Observe your parent closely for signs of improvement and/or worsening. If you see no improvement after a few weeks, *do not* assume that nothing can be done. First, speak to the team caring for your parent; if they can't help and especially if they don't seem to care, seek help elsewhere. If your parent seems to be worsening, notify the nursing or medical staff immediately. Many of the medications used in the treatment of mental disease have strong side effects.

DEMENTIA

If you read this article and learn only one thing let it be the following: *It is not normal to become "senile."*

If someone you love (or for that matter someone you hate) seems to be becoming "senile," that is, if they have severe memory loss or loss of orientation (not knowing where they are, or what day it is, making many mistakes in their work, etc.), it should be investigated. Dementia is such a devastating condition that any possibility for reversibility should be explored. Reversible dementia may be caused by thyroid disease (low or high amounts of thyroid hormones in the blood), vitamin deficiencies (especially B12 and folic acid), or brain disease (e.g., tumors or increased fluid pressure in the brain [hydrocephalus]). All of these must be ruled out before the person is diagnosed as having an irreversible dementia.

Two other important causes of "reversible" dementia should be noted. One is over-medication. Many older people on numerous medications both self-prescribed and prescribed by doctors, become confused, lethargic, seemingly demented. When the medications are adjusted or changed, they improve. Remember—elderly people are very susceptible to the effects of drugs: 1) The body is less able to excrete bodily wastes. The kidneys, although they seem to be functioning perfectly are clearing toxins (poisons) at a much slower rate, so drugs are kept around in the body longer, therefore we need less. 2) Many elderly people receive a number of drugs—because of numerous health problems. 3) It is sometimes easier for a person to take a sleeping pill or a tranquilizer or for a health professional to give one than to deal with the real underlying problem, e.g., depression, anxiety. 4) All drugs have beneficial and negative effects. You can't have one without the other.

Another serious cause of what is called "pseudo-dementia" is depression. Some elderly people, when they become depressed also become withdrawn, become disinterested in life, don't care to talk, or listen, or care for themselves. They can be misperceived as demented.

So, to reiterate, the elderly person who seems to be becoming demented must be investigated—preferably by a geriatric assessment team—for the reversible causes of dementia. If they turn out to have a reversible cause, it is wonderful. But again, to face reality, many causes of dementia are not reversible. One, called multi-infarct dementia, is caused by numerous small strokes. Another, the most common form of dementia, is Alzheimer's Disease. (See also the chapters on dementia.)

DEPRESSION

Depression is a condition characterized by sadness, loss of interest in life, difficulty in sleeping, loss of appetite, feelings of hopelessness, and, when very serious, a desire to commit suicide. It can occur under a number of different situations and, in the elderly, can mistakenly be attributed to "aging."

Prolonged grief. Sometimes the normal grief that occurs after the death of a loved one or another serious loss can go on for a very long time, even years. When it seems that the grief is never-ending and the person does not seem to be regaining at all the joy of living, we call it depression.

Depression *caused by medications of a physical illness.* Certain medications of physical illnesses may cause depression, not because the person is sad due to the problem, but because of a chemical abnormality in the brain caused by the drugs. For example, reserpine is a drug sometimes used for hypertension (high blood pressure). It was used much more frequently until certain people developed depression to the point of suicidal tendencies. Some other hypertension drugs that can cause depression are alpha-methyldopa (Aldomet), and clonidine

(Catapres). Recently, even some diuretics have been reported to cause depression. Diazepam (Valium) and all its relatives can bring out what is called masked depression. They should not be used in the treatment of depression. Hypothyroidism is a classic disease causing depression. Other conditions that can cause depression include Parkinson's Disease, certain cancers, and menopause. When a person becomes depressed, it is very important to rule out these and other medical causes of depression.

Endogenous depression. Essentially, it just happens, out of the blue. Even as a physician, I find this third one hard to accept—that we can just become depressed, out of the blue, as if some inner magical knob is being turned on and off.

When someone becomes depressed, I don't feel good when they are labeled with a diagnosis and treated as if they have a disease. I firmly believe that grief, sadness, anxiety, loneliness, fear, or purposelessness are feelings with which we all must cope at some time in our lives. Treating these feelings with medications may deal with the symptoms, but does not deal with the underlying problems. In fact, particularly in the elderly, drugs can often make matters worse. For example, the older person who feels useless and does little all day long has trouble sleeping at night. The physician prescribes a sleeping pill. The side effects of the pill make the person slightly groggy and a bit forgetful during the day reinforcing the sense of worthlessness and fears about aging, literally making the individual less effective.

As you can see, I don't particularly like medications in the elderly, especially in the areas of mental health. Nevertheless, they do have their place and when used properly, in low doses, for limited periods, can be helpful. Under what circumstances might it be appropriate? In the case of (1) severe depression that seems to come from nowhere and doesn't respond to psychotherapy (i.e., talking, discussion); (2) a prolonged depression that does not respond to therapy; or (3) a "psychotic" depression—an extremely severe depression that includes loss of touch with reality. In these cases a trial of antidepressant medication should be used. The main group of antidepressants are the tricyclic (or tetracyclic) antidepressants, so named because of the appearance of their chemical formula. They include Elavil, Tofranil, Sinequan, and Ludiomil. They act in the brain by attempting to change the levels of certain neurotransmitters, chemicals that send messages in the brain. The theory is that some depressed people have altered levels of these brain messengers and that these altered levels make a person feel depressed. The antidepressant medication tries to restore these levels to normal, and in some people they work very well. In others, they don't seem to work at all (and so far, it's hard to know in advance whom they're going to help). So why not try them on everybody? Because like all medications, they have side effects. In some people, they can (but not necessarily will) increase sleepiness, cause double vision, increase urinary retention (the bladder holds onto its urine and doesn't let it out when it should), or increase the chance of glaucoma in susceptible people. Not all the tricyclic antidepressants have the same degree of this kind of side effect (called anticholinergic side effects). Elavil has the strongest degree of this kind of side effect. In fact, it is so sedating (sleep-inducing) that in small doses, some doctors give it as a sleeping pill. A course I took at Harvard several years ago suggested that it never be used with the elderly. I feel that if it is used, it must be used very carefully.

So if your elderly parent is being started on an antidepressant, it's very important to know the degree of side effects it may cause. If your parent has glaucoma, prostate problems, or loves to read, it's important to notify the physician, as this may affect the choice of drug used.

Antidepressants can take ten days to three weeks to be effective. If your relative has a severe depression not responding to therapy and starts the drugs, give them a try for the full three weeks before giving up on them as hopeless (the drug—not your relative). Dosages, as always in the elderly, are lower than in younger people. The physician often will start at a lower dose and work upward. There are some other antidepressants on the market that are chemically different. They are called monoamine oxidase inhibitors and are used less often because of severe side effects, especially a sudden attack of high blood pressure when certain cheeses or wines are eaten.

What Can You Do as a Daughter?

First, if your parent is grieving, try to be a friend and understand. Be patient, open doors to new experiences and sources of joy, but don't resent it if they are not ready to walk through.

Second, if you suspect a depression, consult a physician or psychiatrist, preferably one working with a geriatric or psycho-geriatric team.

Third, make sure they (the physicians) rule out, through examination, blood tests, and review of medications, the possible physical causes of depression.

Fourth, if they suggest medication, discuss which one, why, and the side effects. Watch closely for positive and negative effects.

Fifth, request psychotherapy in addition to medication.

Sixth, if your parent resists going to a psychiatrist, saying for example, "I'm not crazy," help them understand that it is as much for your need as for theirs that they would be going, that they would be helping with your peace of mind, and share your fears and questions with your parent.

Seventh, if they have to be hospitalized, continue to be your parent's advocate: watch for improvement or worsening in your parent; watch out for over-medication; get the geriatric team involved—sedation and confusion are not necessary side effects. Sometimes with help, the person can be cared for at home—discuss this with your physician.

Good luck. It's not easy. Trust your intuition. Trust yourself as a therapeutic tool—in our own way we can all heal and be healed—allow this process to occur between you and your elderly parent.

I'd like to end with some of the best advice I have ever heard in relation to the issues we have dealt with in this section and to life in general, written by Hillel, a Hebrew philosopher who lived in the first century b.c. He said, "If I am not for myself, who will be for me? If I am only for myself, what am I? If not now, when?"

SUPPORTING
INDEPENDENCE

Helping aging parents maintain some degree of independence in their own homes can involve most, or all, of the activities of daily living including food preparation, monitoring medications, exercise, personal grooming, laundry, and arranging for continuing social contacts. Providing this help necessitates frequent, perhaps daily visits, shopping, transportation, and advocacy during illness and hospitalization. This range of activity can become, in effect, a second (or third) career for the caregiver.

"Research has shown that the amount of time middle-aged women spent providing care increased with age. Women aged 40 to 49 averaged 3 hours weekly; those between the ages of 50 to 59 averaged 15.6 hours weekly of help given; and those who were age 60 and older were giving an average of 22.7 hours a week to their elderly mothers" (E. Shanas, "Older People and Their Families: The New Pioneers," *Journal of Marriage and the Family* 42 (1980):9–15).

Mary Anne describes her caregiving career in detail—the long struggle involved in "keeping a forgetful mother going" after an injury and hospitalization. Jeanne responds with important tips regarding well-being for the caregiver. Her messages are practical and personal, born of her own experience as a caregiver for her dying mother. Sue focuses on the "hospital" experience in particular—one of those life experiences that has the potential for being either truly health-promoting . . . or simply horrendous. Lisa responds directly to Mary Anne's concern about her mother's memory loss in the section entitled "Dementia."

Keeping Mother Going

Mary Anne Montgomery

"Mother, your feet are dragging."

"I know. It's because I'm tired," she explained again.

That foot-dragging dialogue had been played and replayed countless times. I began to feel like a nag. But the shuffling got on my nerves somehow—it seemed so lazy, and it made Mother seem even older than her eighty years.

Could she walk normally if she tried harder, or was this just an inevitable part of aging? Should I remind her, or should I let it go? I often wished I could talk it over with an expert on physical fitness, but I didn't know one. I also wondered how best to handle her increasing forgetfulness.

Still, Mother seemed to get along pretty well. She had moved from another state to be near us, and she liked having her own home nearby. Her apartment complex was built expressly for people aged sixty and over, and it was outfitted with many features to make their lives easier and safer. Mother was still driving and often said she never wanted to give it up. We visited by phone every morning and saw each other two or three times a week. Mother was always with us for Sunday dinner. Quite abruptly, though, our togetherness became a daily necessity. The foot-dragging that had bothered me caused Mother to have a fall that greatly changed our lives. Later, I read in Alex Comfort's *A Good Age* that tripping is the most common cause of falls.

It began with a phone call from the supermarket manager explaining that Mother had "had a little accident." He said, "I think she's more shook and embarrassed than hurt."

Indeed, that seemed to be the case when I got to the store. Mother had apparently tripped on a metal strip across the entryway. That strip was nearly flush with the floor and would not have been an obstacle to the average shopper, but Mother was probably tired that late Friday afternoon. Sitting on a bench inside when I reached her, she said the knee she had landed on wasn't so sore now. She thought she could walk to her car. The manager helped her up and out, and I drove her home and got her settled with an ice pack on a badly bruised knee.

Later that evening, the pain worsened, and Mother could no longer stand. The doctor told her to go to the Emergency Room for x-rays. The ambulance ride with "those nice young men" was Mother's last distinct memory of the first two months of recovery from a fractured leg.

THE TRAUMA OF INJURY

For Mother the fracture was catastrophic. I was appalled that a "minimal fracture" behind the knee could have such a devastating effect on the entire mind and body. Mother seemed like a balloon that had been pricked and lost all its air. She lay, sometimes pale and listless, other times in pain, with periods of confusion, disorientation, and memory loss. I often found myself visiting an eighty-year-old, helpless, sad, whiney child who barely resembled the mother I knew. The brief episodes when she looked at me strangely and didn't recognize me were eerie and frightening.

While I was at a concert one evening, she telephoned from the hospital to ask if I would take her home "from this strange place." My son, Jeff, who answered the phone, was puzzled. I telephoned the hospital when I returned, and the nurse explained that it is not unusual for an older person to become confused and disoriented when she is faced with unfamiliar surroundings and routines.

For me those weeks were full of new experiences, responsibilities, uncertainties, decisions to be made, and always, pressures. The trip to the hospital twice a day left little time or energy for household matters. As one who owned four different books on organizing and using one's time wisely, I couldn't find time to read them; I was swamped with work to be done. The house was a mess. Our beloved twelve-year-old basset hound suddenly developed incontinence problems, creating additional chores. I longed for just one full day at home alone to work and gather my thoughts in peace. Yet I seemed always to be driving—to see Mother, or to do errands for her or for my family of five. The children frequently needed to be chauffeured here and there or to be watched in this school program or that game. With the Christmas shopping season upon us, there were family gifts to be purchased. Mother began to have shopping requests for me, too. The physical demands on my time plus the emotional strains of dealing with an unpredictable and different mother reduced me almost to a state of shock. I was mentally and physically numbed.

Numbness was no help in trying to figure out the complexities of Medicare, doctor, and hospital bills or in making plans for Mother's extended care when I didn't know where to turn for guidance. Her own files and health insurance records were a jumble. The policies seemed to be lost. Household and medical bills arrived at her apartment daily, and I found her checkbook stubs a mystery of incompleteness. Having so many tasks and responsibilities dumped on me all at once was terribly difficult. Not even my husband, Mike, truly understood the enormity of the pressures I felt. (He was busy trying to cope with the children, the meals, and the household work I had neglected.) From way back in my childhood came to mind the cry for rescue: "Mother! Please help me!" But of course it was *my* turn to help Mother.

SUPPORT FOR A DAUGHTER

The reaction of friends to news of Mother's hospitalization was invariably, "Oh, I'm so sorry." They were, but they did not really understand what I was going through. I longed to have someone tell me that she did understand, that she knew things were very difficult for me now. But my situation seemed unique. And the rest of the world appeared engrossed in preparations for the holidays.

Over the previous few months I'd heard of a support group for caregivers of elderly family members. I wanted a source of information on aging; also, what kept popping into my mind was the phrase in the publicity for the group about "non-judgmental support." When I spent so much time with Mother, I neglected the rest of my family, and I felt guilty about it. I felt worn out, pressured, and so inadequate in all my roles. I could really use some support.

I finally made myself telephone the facilitator of the group. She told me a bit about the group and invited me to the meeting that night. As trite as it sounds, when I'd finally decided to attend the meeting I felt a big load lift from my shoulders. I even *ran* up the basement stairs, something I'd lost all energy for in recent weeks.

At the meeting I found the group was, indeed, what I needed. The members were warm and welcoming. Each briefly told her own story of caring for an older relative—they had all been through some very difficult times and had found great support in sharing with one another. There *is* something very healing about being able to tell one's experiences and feelings to kindred souls who have had similar ones.

It's difficult for a tired, pressured, saddened caregiver to view her situation objectively. The caregiver tends to ignore her own needs, and members are good at reminding her that she needs to care for herself, too—so much depends on her own well-being. I will never forget the wonderful respite that the group's Christmas exchange made possible for me. My gift was a purple cloth pouch of herbs and epsom salts to be used for an herb bath. As I soaked and luxuriated in the fragrant steaming water after a grueling day, I realized that this was the first frivolous thing I had done for myself in months. What a joy it was! No tranquilizer could have matched it.

THE TRANSITION

After ten days in the hospital, Mother was moved to a convalescent center where she continued to recuperate and receive intensive physical therapy. Mother was never very happy at the convalescent center, although she knew she could not manage at home. The food was seldom satisfactory to her, and she ate very little. She was weak and tired easily. She developed a bladder infection, and her forgetfulness and confusion persisted. The names of staff and of visitors just did not stay with her, though she recognized family readily. My birthday came during this period, and for the first time in forty-six years, Mother forgot it.

The daily physical therapy was difficult and confusing for Mother. At times she persuaded the aides not to take her there because she was "too awfully tired." The therapist told me that she had difficulty remembering what he told her, and she became upset with herself when she did not do well. She did progress, nevertheless. Six weeks after her fall the splint was removed, the leg was x-rayed and declared ready to bear her full weight. Mother began to walk "normally" again using the walker. She said she had always hated the sight of walkers; now she was forced to use one herself.

Two months after the fracture, we were told abruptly that Mother had reached a therapy plateau. She had been taught all that was prescribed, and though she was in no way independent, Medicare payments for physical therapy could no longer be justified. She now must pay the total cost of her room or find a cheaper place to stay and get therapy. Where would she go? In our own home, we could not manage any lifting—I have chronic shoulder problems, and Mike is troubled by an old back injury. If Mother were to return to her home, she would need someone with her at all times. Someone must walk next to her, lightly holding a safety belt around her rib cage. This security measure was necessary for she was, at times, dangerously unsteady. And how would she get physical therapy?

Mother longed to be in her own home again, and there were points in favor of that. One was our hope that the familiar, secure surroundings of home would relax Mother's mind and ease the confusion and memory problems. Secondly, with someone always with her she would get a great deal more walking practice than she had at the convalescent center. There, except in therapy sessions, Mother was pushed in the wheelchair wherever she need to go. There were simply not enough staff members for someone to accompany her with her walker, either for practice or for necessities. But how could we find a twenty-four-hour helper five days before Christmas? At our weekly meeting someone suggested two possible sources: The Older American's Center in town had a list of people interested in helping the elderly at home. The other source was a referral service for home and health care helpers. They charged a fee for matching patient and helper, after which the helper was paid directly. We decided upon the referral service. Before Mother could leave the convalescent center, though, some preparations were necessary. I needed to learn how to help her walk so that I could show her helpers what to do. Her apartment needed some special equipment and some rearranging, too.

Mother's physical therapist volunteered to train me before Mother left. I watched Bill work with her and the others during two three-hour physical therapy sessions. He coached me quite thoroughly in the mechanics of using the walker, both in ordinary and unusual circumstances. He told me privately that the leg was healed; it was Mother's undependable memory that caused her difficulty in learning to walk again. I came away from the therapy sessions with knowledge and also with gratitude and great respect for Bill's patience and perception.

Bill recommended that we get arms for Mother's toilet and a shower bench so that she would never again need to climb over the side of her tub. Both items have been invaluable. Throw rugs in the apartment were removed, and some of the furniture was taken out or rearranged to make room for the walker. After setting up an extra bed for the helper in her living room, it was time to take Mother home. I stayed with her the first two days and nights. Then the first of our two hired helpers arrived.

The first helper, a college student, was helpful and pleasant. She could stay only a week, and a second helper had been arranged. This was an elderly woman who had been recommended with enthusiasm. Her personality and Mother's did not mesh well, however, especially in the small apartment; she was not as much help as she should have been, either. When the helper developed a severe cough one night and took to her bed to stay, she could no longer stay with Mother. New arrangements were indicated. One good aspect of this turn of events was that Mother perked up and began to take over the role of caregiver for her "helper." This new self-chosen responsibility did more to clear her mind and energize her than anything else. She had earlier decided to be helpless and be waited upon— what I jokingly refer to as her "Queen Elizabeth" role. Now *she* needed to do some helping herself.

Still, Mother could not yet be left alone, and with Christmas vacation well underway, we needed another helper. My ten-year-old daughter came to the rescue. Anne pointed out that she was capable of doing all the things Grandma needed, and we had to admit she was probably right. Mother was walking more surely now, and this loving grandmother-granddaughter combination might be the best possible arrangement.

Anne proved to be an excellent helper. She was responsible, caring, con-scientious, and could cope with what little cooking and dishwashing were necessary. She charmed Mother's neighbors who kindly and quite frequently came to call. And her patience seemed unlimited. Now and then when I become exasperated with the behavior of a tired, cranky Anne, I try to remember the Christmas vacation she chose to spend as her grandmother's helper. No one in the world could have filled the position quite as well at the time.

When school resumed I stayed two or three more days and nights with Mother, and then she seemed ready for a night alone. With some trepidation, I left her after dinner, and she managed quite well. Except for occasional evenings when Anne has spent the night there for fun, Mother has not had an overnight helper since.

Following the doctor's recommendation, a physical therapist from the Public Health Nursing Association came to the apartment to assess Mother's progress and prescribe a home exercise program. Sue became a favorite visitor and her cheerfulness and kindness made the detested exercise regimen as pleasant as possible. (We were grateful that this valuable assistance was paid for by Medicare.) The Public Health Nurse, required to come once a month, was a welcome visitor as well.

The crisis passed. Mother, now eighty-one, has been back in her apartment for several months and is more herself. She is in the midst of a long period of rehabilitation and adjustment to being disabled. I no longer feel acutely overwhelmed, but it seems unlikely that we will return to our more separate lives. Every day at the same time I go over to help Mother, dividing my time and energies between our two households. She continues to use her walker, and I've had to face the fact that she is somewhat mentally impaired as well. Her forgetfulness varies in degree from day to day, sometimes from minute to minute.

THE PERVASIVE FORGETFULNESS

The unpredictability of Mother's mental acuity and memory has been the most difficult thing for me to deal with. So many of her problems in coping with daily life have come from being incapable of remembering accurately, or at all. It must be terrifying for her to be unable, at times, to depend upon her own memory and know-how. Although the crisis of a broken leg made memory problems more acute, I discovered that her difficulties were not new. She had been trying to cover up the forgetfulness for years. There had been signs, but I had ignored or excused them.

Before Mother moved to our town, her occasional lapses in correspondence were one clue. Her letters to me several times a week would abruptly stop for two or three weeks. "I'm sorry, I just lost track of the time," she explained. Then I received occasional letters from her friends, concerned about not hearing from their faithful correspondent for months. This embarrassed Mother. She wrote to them immediately, and I forgot about it.

Another difficulty was Mother's creeping procrastination and inertia over matters of importance. This tendency surfaced when my younger son, John, and I went to her distant home to help with the final packing before her move here. Mother had assured me over a six-month period that she was getting ready by sorting, organizing, and discarding the contents of cupboards, closets, and drawers. When I arrived there two weeks ahead of the movers, however, I found that *nothing* had been done.

We completed the packing, drove two thousand miles, and finally got Mother settled into her new apartment. For weeks she tired quickly, was easily confused, forgetful, and slow to comprehend. I explained it, to her satisfaction and mine, as being the result of the exhausting demands of a major move at age seventy-nine. It continued to be easy to explain and excuse each disability as it presented itself, without ever seeing the total picture: Mother was no longer as mentally capable as she had been. I am still working to fully accept that fact and to lower my expectations for her.

It was in seeing and working with Mother closely each day that I became aware of the many areas of daily life that she was not managing as well as I'd assumed. I had long wondered, for instance, why this excellent cook prepared the same few meals over and over again, never trying anything new. It became apparent, however, that she felt she couldn't cope with the complexities of a new recipe. There was comfort in the same familiar dishes, the same way of doing things. It concerned me, too, that food was burned once a week or so.

I found that bill-paying and the keeping of bank and financial records had not been done carefully for years. Until I was forced to do some of it *for* Mother, I'd had no idea. She had long felt it was bad manners to discuss money matters, and it had not occurred to me that Mother might be having difficulty with her household business. She had been, in her sixties, secretary for one of the ministers in a large metropolitan church, where her major responsibility was to deal with thousands of contributions and tithings. Her personal bill-paying now, however, had become haphazard and her financial records were incomplete.

Mother does still write her own checks. Because she voided a great many checks, we now do the bill-paying together. Our business sessions tire her, so we do only one type of work at a time. It's important not to hurry her and not to "overload her mental circuits."[1]

Mother's sense of time has diminished markedly in recent months. We now have a system to keep track of what day it is. Mother has—and *needs*—three calendars in the living room where she spends most of her time. The most essential of these is the little daily calendar next to the telephone. She flips it to the new day on her way to fix breakfast each morning. Every now and then, though, she is uncertain if she has flipped it over. Then comes the early morning phone call to ask me, with embarrassment, what day it is. Mother even telephoned the city's Weather Line to find out the date, but the recording didn't mention it. (There is a widespread assumption that *everybody* knows what day it is.) That prompted me to write to the automobile dealer who sponsors the telephone weather line. I explained Mother's occasional confusion about date, shared by many elderly people, and told of her unsuccessful attempt to find an answer from his weather line. Would he consider adding the date to his telephone recording? The next day he telephoned to say he thought it was a good idea, and from that day forward the date has been included with the weather information.[2]

The tricks Mother's memory plays are frustrating for us both. In every conversation she asks me to come up with a missing word or an elusive thought which abruptly left her. Sometimes we thoroughly discuss some plans in the morning until we're both satisfied that they're understood, but following her afternoon nap, she has forgotten—entirely or in part. That nap is a great culprit—it's as if that subject on the memory blackboard has been erased, or perhaps smeared beyond recognition by sleep. Mother then telephones me in embarrassment (again) to ask me to explain once more.

In an effort to help, I write down more and more things for Mother on her small daily calendar, or on a yellow card. She doesn't particularly like it, though, and sometimes discourages me from leaving a note—"I'm not *that* far gone!" But she is coming to realize that reminders are necessary.

I wish I could say I never lost patience with my mother. I know she cannot control her memory problem. Yet there are times I am cross with her, to my regret. The cumulative effect of dealing with the forgetfulness and confusion causes my frustration to spill over now and then. And even though I usually manage to stifle impatient thoughts, there is sometimes a sharp edge to my voice. Mother is quick to notice it or to hear the preschool teacher sound of my voice as I go over things very slowly and simply for her. Then she mimics me, and I realize what I was doing. My tone of voice was demeaning. I had forgotten what a narrow line there is between speaking clearly and apparent condescension. When I hear myself sounding like the parent of a stubborn child, I realize it is time to head home to be alone for a few minutes to relax, think through my behavior, and regain perspective.

When I am alone I remind myself that Mother "is *not* being obstinate or doing this intentionally."[3] She cannot help her forgetfulness, and impatience on my part can only be harmful. I feel great love and compassion for this woman who has been a part of my life longer than anyone else in the world. I need only to think, too, of how I would wish to be treated in the same circumstance. In light of Mother's present difficulties, it is not comfortable to remember that she and I were each about the same age when our daughters were born. I am mindful that I'm now setting an example for my own future on down the road.

HELPING MOTHER REMAIN AT HOME

As her only child I am doing my best to enable Mother to remain in her apartment. She loves the relative privacy, and she is surrounded by a lifetime of beloved possessions. This constitutes "home" and security for her as no other place could. But some of the most basic needs—food, cleanliness, medication, and exercise—are not easily met by a disabled older person who lives alone. Through many trials and errors Mike and I have come up with several ideas and techniques that have helped Mother.

Keeping her life simple and peaceful, and sticking to a definite routine, help her days pass fairly smoothly. I'm determined to do *for* her only things that she is unable to do. There are so many things that Mother can no longer do, though, that I find myself helping her in more and more capacities. Every day, as physical therapist, I take a thirty-minute walk with Mother, reminding her gently but again and again, of the various things we were taught by the "official" therapists. Mother has never liked exercise, feeling it is an activity "real ladies" do not indulge in. Being tired is Mother's most common explanation for not doing things—left to follow her own inclination, she would fritter away the time and energy of all her days just "taking it easy," dozing in her chair. Her tendency toward inertia and the procrastination I described earlier are ever present and growing stronger. Consequently, I must be her gentle prod repeatedly, frustrating though it is. *Idleness* in Mother's case quickly encourages weakness of muscle and sluggishness of mental ability. A day off from exercise and walking sets her back several days in strength and endurance.

Also, in the role of practical nurse, I've dealt with such health matters as simplifying the medication routine and safety in showering. It surprised me that Mother was having difficulty keeping her medication straight. We had talked about taking the pills with meals, and one more at bedtime, but she didn't remember all four doses. There were several days of hit-or-miss pill-taking before I realized it was too complex a task for Mother. After many attempts, we found a method that worked for her: Mike stressed the importance of having very simple and precise written instructions for her. On a bright yellow card kept next to the pill containers, I printed simple instructions in clear black letters: "One brown pill *and* one yellow and white capsule with breakfast," and underneath it, "One brown pill *and* one yellow and white capsule with lunch," and so on. Pills are placed in small plastic boxes for each dose: a red box labeled "breakfast," a yellow "lunch" box, green for dinner, and blue for bedtime. Bedtime pills are sometimes forgotten, but this system works most of the time. I am still concerned that Mother have her eight 8-oz. glasses of fluid per day, recommended by the doctor and the Public Health Nurse, Lee. When I am with her, we "enjoy" an 8-oz. glassful together. She is on her own for the rest of them, and I doubt that much more has ever been consumed.

I learned early that the morning hours between 10:00 and 12:00 are our most productive. Mother's body, her mind, and her spirit have been fueled by breakfast, and we can accomplish several tasks together with an 11:00 break for tea. Two mornings a week we begin with her shower, as Lee taught us: a rubber mat inside the tub and one outside reduce the risk of slipping. Mother undresses herself, backs up to the shower bench placed crosswise inside the tub, then sits on it. She turns, carefully lifting one leg, then the other, into the tub. She sits the entire time, facing the shower. The showerhead is a convenient one that may be hand-held or hooked up against the wall. For safety I stay with Mother for the getting in and getting out. The shower and dressing procedures are quite tiring for her, so afterward she usually has something to drink and a cookie to eat. Then we do the leg exercises and the long daily walk.

And, of course, I am Mother's chauffeur, her shopping-list-maker, shopper, and delivery person, her dietician (constantly checking her refrigerator—a forgetful person easily loses track of how long something has been in it), her substitute "meals-on-wheels," and, less frequently, cleaning lady and gardener. It is impossible to carry a watering can with a walker, and the flowers on the balcony are a special joy to Mother. The flowers attract the hummingbirds she loves to watch to a nectar feeder hanging above them. Those tiny birds are the only members of the animal world permitted at the apartments; even other types of bird feeders are forbidden.

RESOURCES AND FAMILY HELP ME COPE

From my support group friends who have aging parents I have learned about several books on aging. I have borrowed some and bought others. The more knowledge I have, the better I am able to handle situations as they come up with Mother. *The 36-Hour Day* has been indispensable in dealing with Mother's forgetfulness.

I recently joined the Duke Alzheimer's Family Support Program.[4] Modest dues help support their research on dementing disorders and their assistance to caregivers. In turn, I receive a newsletter, "The Caregiver," which is full of up-to-date information on dementia, and helpful suggestions for patient care.

I feel very fortunate that my family believes in what I'm doing for Mother. They, too, help her in many ways. Mike helps her indirectly a great deal by listening to my descriptions of problems and challenges with her care, then offering suggestions if I ask—he has a way of getting right to the heart of the matter. This ability seems to come from his logical approach to problem-solving and from his being less emotionally involved—this is my mother, not his, and he is able to stand back and see things more objectively. The children are becoming more self-sufficient at home, and they know that untidiness will persist unless all pitch in to keep the house picked up and clean. Some help more than others. Seventeen-year-old John is exemplary. On his own he often sees that a chore needs doing and does it. How I'll miss him when he goes to college next year. Jeff occasionally goes over to visit Mother, giving me a day off. Everyone misses the fresh-baked loaves of bread or warm cookies that often used to await them at the end of the day, but they are understanding. Even though I return from Mother's during the afternoon, I'm often physically and mentally drained. After a late lunch I put my feet up in the solitude of my bedroom and "recharge my batteries." Thus the afternoons seem to vanish and suddenly it's time to fix dinner. Where did the day go?

JUST FOR ME

When Mother broke her leg it was fortunate that I had not reentered the (paid) working world like so many women I know. I have no idea how we would have managed. Helping Mother is, for me, the right thing to do and the only thing I *could* do. This is not to say that I *love* being a caregiver every single day. There is some sense of obligation to it, and there are times I feel resentful about it.

For over twenty-two years I have been the parent of one or more dependent children. I had begun to think it was time to do some things for myself since I was no longer "on call" for a child during the day. While I methodically began to repaint the rooms of the house and do other badly-needed projects, I started to think ahead to work outside the home. Suddenly, though, another dependent needed my care. Mother's need seemed, at first, a temporary need, but it is apparent now that the dependency is open-ended. My projects have been put on hold.

There is something disturbing about realizing that I am the one and only person who is keeping Mother as "independent" as she is today. I recently read, "What happens to the confused, forgetful person if you, the caregiver are injured or become ill? It is important that you have a plan ready."[5] I have no plan, so I had better make one. Meanwhile, I am looking into the possibility of hiring a college student or two who will spend some hours with Mother twice a week, giving me two days off. The change and variety would be good for both of us.

While I have become interested in the subject of aging and am enthusiastic about my support group, I have been unable to talk much about them with Mother. With her I stress my interest in the group as a source of information and help for us. The idea of my needing *support* would dismay Mother. She really has no idea how much I do to keep her going. Her mind cannot grasp the totality of what I do. She tends to think of me as the dutiful daughter who walks with her and waters her plants once a day. It would never occur to Mother that I devote to her a good half of my working time and energy and a great deal of thought and concern. I mustn't imply that she is ungrateful, for she thanks me over and over for my help, but she is aware only of a job here, a job there. This partial awareness of hers is what keeps us from having the nice spontaneous conversations and sharing times we once had. I do miss those good visits. I miss the mother I always knew, and I miss being myself—my real self—with Mother.

To relieve stress and to avoid burnout these days, I am learning to grab some time just for myself and to do more of the things that I love doing. I'm more and more able to push guilt from my mind at the same time. I know it's important to lessen demands on myself and indulge in some pleasurable activities, or in peace and quiet, for respite. A caregiver who feels refreshed is better able to care for an older relative with patience and good humor.

One thing I've done for myself, of necessity, is to lower my housecleaning standards. The once tidy, well-maintained house now needs rejuvenation—we are healthy, clean, and well-fed, but the house is rarely presentable (by my old standards) to drop-in visitors.

Every day, including Sunday, I enjoy a quiet hour before the rest of the family gets up. After a cup of coffee or two my brain begins to perk, and I have uninterrupted time to write letters or to read books on aging, self-improvement, or whatever I wish. It is an hour I look forward to when I go to bed at night. There will always be some time that's mine alone first thing in the morning.

Someone told me about the benefits of systematic relaxation and recommended a text to read and record on tape.[6] I did record it, adding my own description of a very relaxing beach scene. Whenever I'm going through especially stressful times, I listen to the tape for about twenty minutes, relaxing and imagining myself on that beach. It greatly relieves the teeth-clenching, tightly-wound feelings of tension. Cutting down on caffeine has also helped.

While Mother detests exercise, I feel it's essential. I'd given it up during Mother's early convalescence for lack of time, but it's part of my daily routine now. Stretching and limbering exercises, jogging indoors on a trampoline, and strengthening exercises give me greater energy and endurance.

I love to eat and have always done a lot of cooking. When Mother's crisis was upon us and I had no time to cook, I felt frustration rather than relief. It was then I realized that for me cooking is a pleasure and a need as much as a duty. Consequently, I continue to cook and bake far more than my limited time warrants, and we all seem to benefit. My own diet is well-rounded, low in fat, full of whole grains and fresh vegetables, and low on sugars and sweets.

I can lose myself in music. I go to the opera and often listen to it on records and radio. Certain selections exhilarate, others tranquilize, and I choose to suit my needs. Radio talk shows offer escape, information, and food for thought while I do routine chores at home.

As a year-round feeder of birds, I easily become absorbed in the great variety of feathered beings outside our windows. Guilt feelings still dog me though when I take time off for myself, when I'm not "accomplishing things." Perhaps it's partly because Mother was always a tireless worker who rarely took time for herself until forced to bed with a migraine. It *is* perfectly all right to sit with my feet up for a few minutes and do nothing. It is a "must" after a morning at Mother's. My bedroom becomes my haven, my "decompression chamber."

I try to take each day as it comes, realizing that each one will be different and likely to yield a few unexpected twists. Although Mother is unlikely to improve dramatically, I can certainly make an effort to appreciate and enjoy her good days, while trying not to become frustrated over bad ones. I hope to learn to be easy-going over her frequent repetition. She cannot remember having thanked me ten times for dinner, for instance, but what of it? It is better than mean, unkind words and is just one of those tiresome things I must learn to accept.

It is easy to become wrapped up in duties. I have an enormous sense of time and events moving swiftly yet of having too little time to notice: Anne will be eleven only once; John's senior year in high school is *now;* Jeff may move to another city or place of his own after this year. I want to take time to notice, enjoy, and appreciate, as I'll never be able to recapture these months. The children, too, will never have better opportunities to visit with their gentle octogenarian family member. She loves seeing them, and will probably tell them of her gratitude several times over during each of their visits together.

A LEGACY

I realize that over the last two years my children have become more aware of and even enlightened about the elderly—their needs, their special qualities, their physical abilities or disabilities. The day-to-day involvement of our family in Mother's struggles and failures to remain "independent" has taught them a great deal about sharing, caring, giving, and receiving. They have learned the importance of tact and patience; they see how essential it is that someone who needs help receives it; they're aware that their mere presence can change their grandmother's gloom to cheerfulness. Conversations with her are seldom normal, sprinkled as they are with memory gaps. But the children's patience, understanding, and warmth make her feel loved and at ease.

There have been times when only the children could have provided a particular experience or special help. This summer, in honor of her eighty-second birthday, they gave Mother a small but memorable fireworks show in the backyard. (They understood, too, her need to view it from indoors where there was less noise.) When Mother fell in her apartment and was unable to get to her feet but did reach the telephone, it was John and Jeff to whom she turned for help. "Now, don't tell your mother!" she pleaded. John is her Mr. Fix-it of gadgets and radio and TV. Jeff, our artist, surprised her with a gift of his oil painting of her favorite sunrise view from the balcony windows.

Anne, now 12, whose fuse can be very short when she's thwarted, is able to be calm and patient with her grandmother's forgetfulness, confusion, and snail's-pace walk. A recent telephone conversation following Mother's nap illustrates:

Anne: Oh, hello, Grandma. (Pause)
       No, we aren't coming over to pick you up for dinner today. That will be on Saturday. (Pause)
       Today is Thursday, Grandma. (Pause)
       No, we won't pick you up tomorrow, either. Tomorrow is Friday. (Pause)
       Today is *Thursday,* Grandma. Better turn your calendar back to Thursday. (Pause)
       Does it say "Thursday" now? Good. You're welcome. Good-bye.

How glad I was that Anne answered the telephone. My exasperation would probably have surfaced in discussing the date mix-up we'd encountered countless times before.

Mother has no idea that I've *hired* Anne for a token sum to substitute for me at her place twice a week this summer. Anne chats with Mother, waters her geraniums, takes the daily walk with her, and sometimes has lunch and a game of double solitaire. It is a great help to me to be freed to work at home while they're together, and Mother treasures these visits. The routine is sometimes tiresome for my active daughter, but she doesn't reveal her boredom to Mother. I tell her that I understand her feelings, and that I too sometimes feel restless and impatient when I'm helping Mother. But I stress the importance of doing things slowly and calmly with someone who's forgetful like Mother, and Anne feels good about handling this situation successfully.

I feel quite certain that these years of active involvement with Mother will help my children to become adults who will not ignore the needs of our growing elderly population. Most people seldom think about aging until their parents begin to show signs of growing old. I know that my children have become familiar with older people and their needs; I'm hopeful that they will be sensitive to these needs for many years to come.

REFERENCES

1. Nancy L., Mace, and Peter V. Rabins, *The 36-Hour Day* (Baltimore: The Johns Hopkins University Press, 1981), 117.

2. Weatherline, Inc. "Management Agent for U.S. Weathercasts," 12119 St. Charles Rock Rd., St. Louis, MO 63044.

3. Mace and Rabins, *36-Hour Day,* 27.

4. Duke Alzheimer's Family Support Program, Box 2914, Duke Medical Center, Durham, NC 27710. Current Annual Dues: $10.00.

5. Mace and Rabins, *36-Hour Day,* 125.

6. Barbara Powell, *Overcoming Shyness* (New York: McGraw-Hill, 1976).

RECOMMENDED READINGS

Bloomfield, Harold H., with Leonard Felder. *Making Peace with Your Parents.* New York: Random House, 1983.

Briggs, Dorothy Corkille. *Celebrate Your Self.* Garden City, NY: Doubleday, 1977.

Budoff, Penny Wise. *No More Hot Flashes.* New York: G. P. Putnam's Sons, 1983.

Comfort, Alex. *A Good Age.* New York: Crown, 1976.

Kenney, James, and Stephen Spicer. *Caring for Your Aging Parent: A Practical Guide to the Challenges, the Choices.* Cincinnati: St. Anthony Messenger Press, 1984.

Levy, Judith. *Grandmother Remembers.* New York: Stewart, Tabori & Chang, 1983.

Silverstone, Barbara, and Helen Kandel Hyman. *You and Your Aging Parent: The Modern Family's Guide to Emotional, Physical and Financial Problems.* Rev. and enl. ed. New York: Pantheon, 1982.

Stern, Bert, and Laurence D. Chilnick. *The Pill Book.* 3d rev. ed. New York: Bantam Books, 1986.

Stern, Edith M., and Mabel Ross. *You and Your Aging Parents.* New York: Crown, 1965.

Caregiver Well-Being: My Mother's Daughter

Jeanne Beckwith

When approached to write this article, I was not convinced that it was an entirely appropriate thing for me to do, nor was it something that was likely to make me very happy. My mother was very ill and threatening me daily with her death. This is not a very kind thing to say, but that was how I felt. I didn't know if I would survive the test of taking care of her in her final months. I was an unlikely candidate for the task of writing an article on survival tactics for caregivers. Yet, I was my mother's daughter, and despite her tendency to martyrdom, her gloomy predictions about life, and her dim view of my potential as a human being, she loved fiercely, laughed easily, and made it to age eighty-one. She must have been doing something right. Maybe she has passed that secret along to me.

There is no one particular age when we can expect to become caregivers to our parents. It is not a developmental stage. Yet, no matter when it occurs, we can expect to be going through some transitional stage of our own. In my case I was coming up on my fortieth birthday. My mother was eighty-one. She was facing death. I was stepping into the second half of my life. Just the idea of that alone was stress enough, or so it seemed. The years after we turn forty are a difficult time of transition in anyone's life. Change always brings some kind of stress. In our forties we begin to face changes in our bodies and in the way we relate to those around us. Our children are growing up and away from us. Our sexuality takes on a different significance. The dreams we had have either come true, and in the truth of being have ceased to be goals or were not quite what we had

Jeanne Beckwith, MA, a professional playwright with several productions behind her, blends her unique writing ability with personal experience as a caregiver and professional experience as an educator in the field of mental health. She is currently pursuing a Master's Degree in Fine Arts at the University of Georgia, Athens.

thought they would be, or perhaps they have been shattered by the vagaries of time and chance. We begin to be frightened at the prospect of our own mortality. We wonder about our limits. We long for new dreams and work to infuse our lives with meaning. It is little wonder that the added strain of tending to the daily needs of someone else, as Mary Anne describes, can test our patience and bring us to the edge of illness.

Exhaustion and fatigue are sure symptoms of stress. The caregiver may have no sense of rest even upon awakening. Listening in the night, disturbed sleeping arrangements, conflicts in schedule, and other changes in our normal patterns can cause us to feel abnormally tired. Often the caregiver is unable to shake a cold and is subject to flare-ups of chronic illnesses, headaches, gastrointestinal disorders, depression, and weight loss or gain.

Normally talkative and cheerful persons can become silent and taciturn. The easy-going become quick to anger and are easily irritated. This is particularly bothersome because the episodes of anger can lead to increased feelings of guilt. Trusting individuals can become suspicious and wary. We may start to believe that others have no regard for what is being done or think more could be done. This even extends to strangers. I was sure that the interviewer from the Area Agency on Aging thought I was exaggerating about the situation and secretly thought me selfish for having asked for help.

The stressed caregiver is also particularly vulnerable to chemical abuse. Our society and culture often promotes the use of chemicals as a stress reliever, and unfortunately there are doctors who are all too willing to prescribe tranquilizers for a situation that they cannot otherwise cure.

New ideas or change become stressful in and of themselves. We have had enough changes! our psyches seem to scream. Even the suggestion that there are alternatives to the present situation may be viewed as threatening, if not impossible. We can perceive no other options for ourselves and therefore feel left without a choice. I know that I hated all of the alternatives that were suggested to me. Didn't anyone understand that I just wanted my mother back? Why did they keep offering me solutions?

Hardest of all in this process was allowing it to be, and then treating it as normal. I wanted to shrink from the whole thing. Whenever my mother talked about dying, I would get a little crazy. I was sure she was just doing it to get at me. Hadn't she done everything she could to achieve that goal? I would refuse to discuss it. I would say that I knew she would live forever, so we should not worry about it. But we did.

Of course in my heart, I was afraid she would live forever, that there was no end to the situation. She wouldn't, she couldn't die. But I would catch myself scanning the obituaries in the paper each night noticing the ages of those who had gone on, calculating where my mother fit in with the statistics. I think she was ready to die. I wanted to carry on the struggle. I didn't understand that my struggle was not hers, that I wasn't ready to die, but that that didn't mean she couldn't.

My situation was unique to my mother and me, as is that of each reader. Our parents go and die on us (How dare they?) at almost any stage of life, and the parent-child relationship is forged from two unique personalities in harmony or at odds since the birth process. I have tried to speak to all of you, and often I have been speaking to myself. Together perhaps, we can find a way to keep ourselves together and survive a little longer.

Although survival, I must say, is not the exact word I would use. If we are still alive, then we survive, but sometimes I ask myself, can I call this living? Often it is not quite what I had in mind. Still, it came as a revelation to me as I watched my mother die that none of this had been quite what she had had in mind either. I think she was a woman raised to believe in miracles—in happy endings. Her life had been a catalogue of misfortune and unhappiness (God, didn't I hear about it often enough), as well as a few good times. And she kept looking forward to the good times as if they were a gift from heaven to make it all worthwhile. Maybe she was right. But I don't think so, not entirely. If our lives are to have power, we must have more than a positive attitude. I don't know exactly how to explain this, but the whole positive attitude thing implies a belief in the negatives of life and in the struggle that must take place to overcome them. It is based upon some notion that life is a balance of accounts. Life isn't a balance of accounts. What it is, is sometimes hard, sometimes easy. What it can't be, is a lie. When we base our existence on half truths and fairy tales, we give up our hope of being real. To really live we have to tell the truth—not brutally and not without thought. This is especially difficult in a society that teaches us to cover up the truth, paint it over, pretty it up. More often then not, we are rewarded when we deny our feelings. What good are feelings anyway? You can't buy them—not really. As for trust, the child of truth, it is feared. I remember a fable my mother used to tell me that ended with the moral: Don't trust anyone. What about yourself? If I say nothing else in these pages, I hope I get across the idea that you have to trust yourself. Then you won't be afraid to feel the truth. For telling the truth about things will help you get on with life. The parent you are protecting, even your children, deserve to be told the truth. If something is wrong in your life or in the world, don't try to cover it up. You can judge if something is beyond their understanding, but don't try to deny what is there in front of their eyes. Besides, in lying to them, you lie to yourself. You make it easier to live with myths.

I gained fifteen pounds while my mother was with me. Stress and nerves played a part—perhaps. I think it was more due to my own dysfunctional belief system. You see, the kitchen for some reason was the only place in my house where my mother would not venture. It was the only place I could go and be sure that she wouldn't follow. And I felt bad about going there. Rationally, I could understand that I needed time away from her even within the same house, but could I make myself sit and read or write or rest? No, I had to cook. It was a kitchen, wasn't it? I needed a justification for going there that could not include my need to be alone. I didn't accept it. I got out during the day. I saw my friends. It was unkind of me to hide away from her unless. . . . So I baked and cooked. Unfortunately, even though I could say that this was done in order to please my mother—to offer her something different to eat, something she might consider eating—it wasn't true. My mother didn't care about food anymore. She moved food around on her plate, slipped it into a napkin, pretended to chew, but she did not eat. So I did. I couldn't let food go to waste could I? I shudder to imagine just how many chocolate chip cookies and chicken casseroles found their way onto my thighs and backside. I struggle now to make them go away. I worry that I will have a heart attack or that my arteries are being eaten away. I ask you, is this the behavior of a rational human being?

But are we rational? We like to think we are. We make a game of it. Next time you are on a cross-country trip and see something unusual, catch yourself trying to explain it away, miles after it has disappeared, until you come up with a logical explanation—one that, of course, by its very nature is based on limited facts now impossible to prove. I think that's what has been happening our whole lives. It is comforting to have explanations to compartmentalize life, to indulge in minor philosophy in the kitchens of our soul. The truth is that we don't need reasons. We block ourselves by always searching for the logical thing to do, justifying what we have already done, when most often, if we are honest, we do the things we do because they seem to be a good idea at the time.

Since my mother's death, I have been dreaming about her constantly. In these dreams I am confronted by her return from the grave. I awake upset and appalled by the anger expressed through the dreams. Well, I tell myself, I was often angry with her in life, why not in death? Yet, like all "good" daughters of our culture, I feel guilty and ashamed that I was not and am not a perfect caregiver. During the last year of her life I watched her getting more and more frail and ultimately confused. Maybe that is part of my frustration now. While she and I argued most of our lives together over who or what we thought the other should be, at the end it was impossible to fight her. She couldn't fight back. Not that she didn't try to fight with me. During the time she finally agreed (Agreed? I dragged her kicking and screaming.) to live with me, she was alternately disagreeable and pathetic. I don't know which was worse. I was determined, however, not to fight with her. So I spent a lot of time being mad at systems—the nursing homes, the welfare office, the federal government, the entire medical profession. It was a fertile ground for all the hurt and upset I had festering within, especially since none of these systems was perfect and my complaints were in many ways legitimate. I wonder, though, how much of the anger I unloaded in their direction was anger I couldn't direct toward my mother for fear of unleashing something I couldn't control against this woman whom I happened to like. This woman who made me crazy for thirty-nine years. This woman I was furious with for dying.

After all, I only wanted her well and living in her little house doing exactly what she had always done—calling me periodically to remind me that I hadn't turned out at all like what she had thought would be best but that she continued to love me anyway. I often wondered what the ideal daughter would have been like. During one of our battles years ago when I had gone off to someplace undesirable in search of something inappropriate, I had yelled at her to tell me what she wanted me to be and I would pretend to be it! She had only shook her head. Sadly enough now, I think she really only wanted me to be happy and in her experience had no way to teach me how.

How many of us struggle our entire lives just to get through? How much do we hide and deny? How much that could perhaps be fixed if we just had the ability to take it out and see it in the light? I think that is what we must do if we are to survive whatever difficulties come our way in life, most especially the difficulty of dealing with our aged parents. It is the only way to come out on the other side as better individuals—stronger maybe—as people who can learn how to be happy by not just accepting life's hassles but by burning them into the very experience needed to find the way to the next arena of our lives. And to do this it is necessary to let a lot of ideas die first—or at the least be relegated to the bottom of our basket of survival tricks.

This is not easy. If it were, the mental health professionals would soon run out of things to do. How we see ourselves—the rules we have about the way we live, the way we act—this is our sense of self and how we fit that self into the world around us. We developed these ideas, these patterns, in order to survive, and now we may find them getting in the way of our survival.

Our society, churches, and families all contribute to the collection of ideas and rules that determine how we move about in the world, the kinds of roles we adopt, the attitudes we espouse. In taking care of our elderly parents, these habits of thought and belief can make the difference in how well we cope with the stresses all around us. One of the ironies of this is that the parents we are caring for probably forged those ideas in us and are just as vulnerable to the kinds of problems they create as we are. Also compounding this problem is the fact that some of the best and noblest visions we have for mankind are involved with ideas that may sound terrific but in practice can make us into physical and sometimes mental wrecks.

Dedicated individuals are the backbone of our society. They are people with vision, people with goals. While dedication may be a virtue in and of itself, it can get us into trouble. The dedicated caregiver has a tendency to take on too much for too long, too intensely. This will be true in the parent-child relationship as well as most other aspects of their lives. Dedicated individuals are apt to sublimate their own needs to those of the "cause." If the "cause" happens to be a parent, a child, a church, or a bridge club, this person will push himself or herself to the burnout level.

Women who are caregivers sometimes neglect to develop other aspects of their lives. The world outside the caregiving situation can be frightening, or perhaps there has been a history or pattern of unsatisfactory experiences. The care of the aging parent can become a substitute for social or vocational achievements—a substitute focus.

I don't know where I could come up with studies or statistics to back up the next statement, but I would bet a lot of money that it's true. Almost every person reading this article has a need to be in control. Even the most self-denying of us has probably developed that habit of unselfishness in order to have a sense that we are in control of things and of others. "See how much I give? How much I sacrifice? How could you possibly thwart someone as wonderful as I?" A lot of us learned this lesson remarkably well right at our parent's knee. We have a need to prove that no one else can do anything as well as we can. Unfortunately, this has the effect of producing a cynical attitude among other members of the family (who know in their hearts that they are the ones with all the answers). These others who could be helping out (thus opening themselves up to the possibility of not measuring up) more often end up distancing themselves from the situation. All this does is reinforce the caregiver's belief that "no one else cares as much as I do."

People are so silly. We want to be perfect. We want to be right. We want to be so many things that are beyond our humanity and think that we should be rewarded for it. I am always amazed when I have driven my point home—proven the validity of my ideas, demonstrated beyond all doubt what a clever, dedicated, honest, caring, and superlative creature I am—to find out that nobody wants to know and that it didn't make any difference anyway. We are going to be dead for a ridiculously long period of time. Couldn't we spend less time trying to be right and more time dancing? All caregivers need to give up the notion that they have or can come up with the formula for success. They will be happier immediately. If only we can learn to trust ourselves to be well-meaning, trust ourselves to be loving and worthy of love, trust ourselves to do the best we can. We are what we are. We can take our lives as a series of mistakes and problems or choose to see it in terms of alternatives and solutions that work or don't work. If they don't work, look for others.

Of course, it matters that you do your best to keep your parents safe and cared for, but you have to keep remembering who you are in this relationship. You are their child and will always be their child. Even when my mother could no longer remember where she had seen me before, I knew I was her daughter. And whatever our parents' problems might have been, whatever their belief systems were composed of, whatever their limitations, they had a child once, and they wanted that child to be happy, to be whole. Maybe they didn't know how to say it and had no more idea than we do of how to make it happen, but in their hearts they wanted it. I don't ascribe to the belief that we owe our parents, just because they are our parents. As usual, life is not a balance of accounts, it doesn't even out. Yet, I think that it is alright to owe them this—to be whole, to be fine, to laugh and cry and search for your dignity and your strength.

SPEAK UP FOR YOURSELF

Whether you are dealing with the doctor, your family or your parent, remember that your opinion is as valid as anyone else's. There are a lot of apparent facts floating around that we would be fools not to recognize, but our feelings, our beliefs, our ideas are important; you have a right to have them. If you find that the people you are with deny your right to have your own opinions, then get away from them. Choose other experts, other friends. It's alright if they disagree with you, but don't let them put you down or punish you for it. And while you're at it *don't put yourself down*. No one is perfect. You must forgive yourself for making mistakes. And learn to accept compliments.

MAKE YOUR OWN DECISIONS

And let your parents make theirs too, if they are competent. Thinking for yourself means you are an active participant in your own life. It puts some of those good times within your reach.

BELIEVE IN YOURSELF

Don't wait for someone else to tell you that you count. Some of your own unfinished business with your parents that is getting in the way of what you need to do for them now may be your bitterness that they never believed in you. So what? They probably didn't know what they believed in. I felt sorry for myself because my mother had never said I was good at anything, until, in talking to another family member, I learned that she had grown up in a culture with a superstition that saying nice things about people you loved might bring harm to them—might expose them through your pride to the evil eye. Good heavens, the woman was protecting me! So I spent a lot of time whining about something that didn't mean what I thought it did. Don't waste any more time waiting for someone else to give validity to your life. Even if someone does come along, you will be so used to your waiting that you may not take this person seriously unless you have already decided to believe in yourself.

BE ALL THAT YOU CAN BE

Take some risks. Don't rely on others to do things for you that you can do yourself. Maybe they could have done it better, but you may be passing up an opportunity to learn and grow.

TEND TO YOUR NEEDS

You cannot take care of others if you don't take care of yourself. If you feel unfulfilled, unfinished, you will have little of any value to give to others and may end up resenting the depletion of your limited resources.

BE PROUD OF YOURSELF

You are unique, and by your very existence you have worth. You are only human, but that implies the possession of much that is great, albeit problematic.

LET GO OF THE PAST

An all-consuming absorption with the past will have a negative influence on your current functioning. What once existed between your parents and yourself doesn't have to define your relationship with them today. So many times we are victims of a belief that simply because something was once true it will always be true. It is important that some aspects of our past be dealt with if we are to come to terms with the present situation. If a past quarrel or situation can be resolved, resolve it. Otherwise let it go. It's like my history of fighting with my mother; of needing to win. There is no way to win and besides, what would be the triumph in defeating a frail, forgetful, old woman?

ACCEPT WHAT IS

We make ourselves miserable more often than not by clinging to the belief that things should be different from the way they are. So instead of dealing with the present situation, we spin our wheels, stuck and ineffectual, because we want what is not possible—we want what is not.

TAKE LOVE AS YOU FIND IT

We want so much to be loved, and that's okay; it's nice to be loved if it is by the right people for the right reasons. Qualifiers. We qualify love and by doing so we rid it of its significance for us. The ability to love us is something we cannot force upon those around us. We are even less able to make them love us the way we want. We must take love where we find it and on its own terms. Flexibility is an important aspect in life. Be flexible about love. It won't come in precisely the form we think it should, so it's better to adapt ourselves to the shape it does take.

FIND SUPPORT SYSTEMS

Try to be with other people as often as you can. Choose people who know you well and care about you. If your parent doesn't know you any more, this is more necessary than ever. He or she may have gone on a separate journey that you cannot be a part of. Don't make yourself sick with loneliness when there are people around who need you as much as you need them. If you don't feel you have anyone in your immediate family or circle to turn to, join support groups, go to educational functions. If you can't be doing anything else you can be learning.

The process of education is vitally important to you at this point in your life. And not simply because knowing more about your parent's problem, or the resources available, will help you to cope more effectively. Don't get me wrong, I think those are important things. But this is a time when things around you are ending. Avenues are closing down. You are constantly being reminded of limits. It is important that you make the attempt to stretch yourself. What you learn is important and helpful. The fact that you can learn it—the process of learning it—will strengthen your whole being.

LOOK WITHIN

This is a time for self examination. Perhaps no other experience in our lives can serve as well to lay our lives out in front of us as the care of our parents. Our childhood is so wrapped up in these people. It stretches out behind us bound in vivid pictures of a time that will not come again and of the experience that brought us where we are today. We will find ourselves remembering details that had been buried, details that give us clues to our strengths and weaknesses, patterns that were born so long ago but that continue to affect our present situation.

Likewise, the future is there if we are brave enough to face it. Our parents' aging is part of an inevitable process that we too in time will have to experience. We come face to face with death. We always knew that sometime we would die, but did we ever really believe it?

Now is our opportunity to listen to our hearts and recognize just who we have always been—good-hearted people with the courage needed to live gracefully for as long as we can and leave our own sons and daughters with a guide for how to care for us and how to let us die.

Support for a Hospitalized Parent

Sue Morrissey

Admitting your parents to a hospital is something you may or may not dread. Some people view hospitalization as a period of relief from the daily responsibilities of parent care. Hospitalization should not be viewed as a panacea, although it may give you some much-needed rest. Neither should it be dreaded as "the beginning of the end." Regardless of how you view the prospect of hospitalization for your aged parent, there are a number of potential pitfalls in hospitalizing an elderly person. Some of these pitfalls will be discussed in this chapter. Suggestions will be offered on how to minimize the dangers and maximize the benefits of your parent's hospitalization for both you and your parent.

ADVANCE PLANNING

You may hope you will never have to hospitalize your parents, but there is a very real possibility that you will find it necessary to do so at some time, either for illness or injury. As Mary Anne points out, her mother's injury, though "minimal," triggered a sudden hospitalization. No matter how you feel about the hospitalization, planning ahead can position you to negotiate the system more effectively. Advance planning includes building a relationship with your parent's attending physician and developing relationships with hospital personnel.

Sue Morrissey, DNS, RN, held staff and administrative nursing positions in hospitals for over twenty-five years. At present she is an Assistant Professor in the Primary Health Care Nursing Department at Indiana University School of Nursing (Indianapolis) and the project director for the Adult/Gerontology Nurse Practitioner program.

74

The Physician

The physician needs to be a person with whom your parent feels comfortable and in whom both of you have confidence. To maintain autonomy as much as possible, your parent needs to be involved in the decision regarding a physician. However, sooner or later you may have to assume at least some responsibility for your parent's care. It is advisable that you get to know the physician and be certain he or she understands what you expect in the way of information and care.

Your parent may or may not have had a physician for a long time, or at least prior to your assuming caregiver responsibility. Several factors should be considered when deciding to retain a physician or when choosing a replacement. One consideration is whether your and your parent's view of what is an appropriate approach to caring for your parent is compatible with the physician's approach to caring for elderly people. Issues that you and/or your parent should discuss with the physician include the physician's approach to a "symptom" in an elderly person. While you and your parent will want a concerned investigation of symptoms, does this physician believe that all symptoms should be explored to determine the cause no matter what the discomfort or risk to an elderly person? For elderly people, particularly frail elderly, the benefits of possible tests and treatments should be weighed against the risk and discomfort to the individual of that particular test, treatment, medicine, or operation. One example would be an x-ray that involved laxatives and enemas as part of the preparation. If the only treatment for the suspected cause is a serious operation, which your parent is too frail to tolerate, why perform the test? If the test is designed to identify a cause that cannot be treated or that may involve treatment that your parent does not want, why put the patient through the inconvenience and the possibility of adverse reactions?

If you and your parent want to be active participants in your parent's care, it is important that you, your parent, and the physician understand that you want to be informed. Being informed means that you want to be told what the physician is planning for your parent, why, what might be the problem, what the options are, and the risk and benefits of a particular course of action. The very nature of a physician's training may lead to a somewhat autocratic approach in planning and decision-making.

A physician who dismisses an elderly person's symptoms and complaints as due to "your age" is to be avoided. This response by their physician is frequently reported to me by my elderly clients. Some older people change physicians in an effort to find someone who will listen to them. Aging is a process about which we know relatively little. If your parent has a complaint or symptom that you think should be investigated, be persistent.

Even worse than ignoring the complaint is giving the old person something for her (this happens most often to women) nerves. Beware of sleeping medications and "nerve" medications for elderly, which would include those to tranquilize or lessen anxiety. Any symptoms or changes in behavior that develop in an older person on these medications should be attributed to the medication until proved otherwise and should be reported to the physician who ordered the medication.

If you want to be involved in this process of planning and have selected a physician who believes that all decisions should be made by the physician, you are headed for trouble, misunderstanding, frustration, anger, and a break-down in communications. This does not benefit you, your parent, or the physician. Mutual respect and a willingness to listen on the part of all concerned parties is an ideal worth striving for in your relationship with a physician.

Prior to selecting a physician for your parent (or before changing physicians), you need to find out to which hospital the physician has admitting privileges. For example, if the physician's office happens to be midway between your home and the hospital where he would admit your parent, this may make a trip to the office convenient for you but visiting your hospitalized parent very inconvenient. The patient/family relationship with the physician is more important, but convenience is a consideration.

I have indicated that an open, honest, and information-sharing relationship should be established with the physician because I believe this is very important in assuring your involvement in your parent's care. Your parent may not see this as so important. Many older people accept the notion that the "doctor knows best." He or she has a great deal of knowledge, but you, the caregiver, probably know your parent better than anyone else. I believe your parent will benefit from your input into treatment and care during hospitalization.

You should also have a voice in the decision to hospitalize. Many tests can be done on an outpatient basis. Some surgical procedures can also be performed and your parent discharged on the same day. The risks of confusion or some "misadventure" during hospitalization are high enough that the decision to hospitalize should not be made lightly. Your physician needs to know you feel this way and will not know unless you and/or your parent make your wishes clear.

HOSPITAL PERSONNEL

The other part of planning ahead is cultivating contacts within the hospital where your parent may someday be admitted. This means that you keep a mental note, if not a written one, of the people you know who work in the hospital or who have relatives who work in the hospital where your parent would be admitted. It never hurts to use all your resources. I have relatives who did this very effectively. For example, an aunt whom I had not seen since I was five years old was admitted to the hospital where I worked. Within twenty-four hours she managed to let me know that she was there. I, of course, visited her regularly. I will not say that my regular visits affected her care in any way, but they certainly did not hurt. A cousin of my father's had a "routine" when she was admitted to the hospital where I worked. As she came through the door of the emergency room, usually on an ambulance stretcher, she announced to anyone within earshot that she was my cousin. She perceived that this somehow gave her special status, since I was a supervisor at the time. Again, it certainly did not hurt. I visited her regularly and took an interest in her care. People whom you know that work in a hospital can probably be counted on to show a similar interest in your parent. Depending on their position, "inside contacts" may be able to give you some hints on negotiating the system in a particular hospital.

ADMITTING YOUR PARENT TO THE HOSPITAL

You can ease the admission process by keeping a record of your parent's health history. As people get older their history frequently becomes long and it is difficult to remember dates, places of hospitalization, and attending physicians. Keeping your own record of this information can speed this part of the admission process. You will also need your parent's Medicare, Medicaid, or supplementary insurance cards.

On admission to the hospital and/or admission to the nursing unit of the hospital the patient is usually asked to give extensive information. It is better to allow your parent to give as much as possible of the required information. Sometimes nurses are "turned off" by relatives who constantly interrupt with additions or corrections. Don't be offended if you are asked to leave the room while the nurse questions your parent and takes what is often referred to as a nursing history. The nurse needs to establish a relationship with your parent and learn your parent's view of needs and symptoms. This is often best accomplished by a private interview. On the other hand, the nurse may ignore your parent and ask you to be the information giver. It then becomes your responsibility to say (if appropriate) that your parent can give the information.

Your responsibility is to make sure that the nursing staff and the physician have the information they need to take care of your parent. Necessary information includes: allergies (food and drug), current medications, medications that your parent took in the past five years, any food idiosyncrasies, or a recent death of spouse. This is a good time to indicate if your parent needs any help with eating and how much assistance is needed (e.g., unable to cut meat, or to hold a glass). You also need to alert the nursing staff to your parent's need for assistance in getting up or walking. This includes problems with dizziness and the need for a cane or walker. Patients are sometimes "selective" in the kinds of information they choose to give the nurse. I have had patients deny any chronic illnesses only to discover later, in one instance, that the person was a diabetic and had been taking insulin for several years.

The patient, the family, and the nursing staff may not have similar ideas of what is important. It is better to give too much information rather than too little. If the nurse does not consider the information important she may ignore it. If you consider the information important make sure that everyone understands the importance. Sometimes just knowing what kinds of medication your parent is taking, and when, may not indicate the importance of the medication. An example of this would be an elderly person who had parathyroid surgery at some time in the past and required large doses of calcium each day. Omission of this medication would be very dangerous. If the nurse does not understand why your parent is getting the calcium she may interpret it as being to prevent or minimize osteoporosis and not attach much importance to giving the calcium regularly. Other information that should be shared with the nursing staff includes any problems with vision and hearing. It is also important to tell the nurses your parent's preferences regarding position in bed if your parent cannot give this information.

Do not depend on the physician to share all required information about your parent. The physician does not have your parent's record either at home (if contacted there) or at the hospital. It is not realistic to expect a physician to remember everything about your parent even if the physician has cared for your parent for a number of years. The physician has also been caring for a number of other people for years.

Do Not Resuscitate Order

When your parent is admitted to the hospital, or shortly thereafter, you may be asked by the physician or by one of the nurses if you want your parent resuscitated should this become necessary (that is, should heartbeat or breathing stop). This request is routine in some hospitals for all persons over a given age and may be completely unrelated to your parent's condition.

Some parents may have prepared a document called a "living will" or may have discussed such issues ahead of time with their children. In that case, responding to the hospital's question will be greatly simplified. If the hospital does not ask, and your parent has clearly expressed preferences in this matter, you will want to convey that to the staff and to the physician.

This is a difficult issue to discuss with loved ones, however, and it may not yet have been approached by anyone in the family. It is certainly easier to have discussed the matter beforehand rather than in the midst of crisis. If that is not the case, however, in most instances you do not need to respond to the query immediately, allowing you some time to seek support from your family and counsel from the physician and other professionals. For further information regarding "do not resuscitate" or "no code" orders, see the chapter "Decision-Making in Health Care."

ADVOCACY

Your most important role while your parent is in the hospital is to look out for what you believe to be your parent's best interests or what you think your parent would want. Advocacy includes monitoring the care your parent is receiving, diet, medications, and tests. You will also want to check drainage tubes to be sure they are draining and note if intravenous fluids or tube feedings are dripping. Anything that is not working as you expect should be reported immediately. Be sure the suspected problem is checked and corrected before you leave. As an advocate, you must also find out if your parent is receiving medication that was taken prior to admission, and if not, to learn the reason for the change. You may have to talk to the nurse or dietition about the diet your parent is getting, particularly if your parent is not eating very well. Sometimes patients are left on liquid diets longer than necessary due to an oversight. *Be prepared to ask questions.* You need to learn what tests are being ordered, their purpose, and how strenuous they are going to be for an old person. Many procedures require harsh laxatives and repeated enemas as part of the preparation. At a time when bowel control may already be diminished, laxatives and enemas increase the likelihood of accidents. Accidents decrease your parent's self-esteem and sense of control. Sometimes alternative procedures are available that will not be so strenuous. Occasionally the preparation for the test can be modified.

GETTING INFORMATION

In order to perform your advocacy role effectively, you need to be as informed as possible. At the time your parent is admitted to the hospital, it is useful to find out from the nurse who admits your parent whether or not this particular hospital uses a team or primary care approach to providing nursing care. If the facility uses primary care, this means that your parent's care will be assigned to one particular nurse. Other nurses may provide the actual care from time to time but one person is assigned responsibility for planning that care. You need to find out who this nurse is and establish a relationship with her (or him) as early as possible in your parent's hospitalization. The person who is responsible for your parent's care is also accountable for much of that care and can be a source of needed information. If a team approach is used on the nursing unit, you will need to identify the leader of the team that is responsible for your parent. The nurse responsible for managing the unit, department, or floor may be called "head nurse," or "nurse manager," or a similar title, and you will want to know that person also. It would be a good idea to introduce yourself. Another staff member who is vital to the team, knowledgeable about the unit, floor, or department, and can provide you with helpful information, is the ward secretary, or ward clerk.

One source of information you may find helpful is your parent's chart. Most hospitals require a physician's order to permit you to read the chart. From the chart you can learn what medicine your parent is getting, what tests are ordered, and how the doctor views your parent's condition as well as his plans for your parent. Ask the nurse or doctor to explain anything you don't understand.

Regular contact with your parent's physician is a necessity while your parent is in the hospital. Sometimes it is difficult to contact a physician. One strategy is to call from your parent's room as soon as you arrive and ask that the doctor return your call. Some physicians return calls after office hours. If your physician does this, you will need to leave a number where you can be reached at that time. Asking the nurses when your parent's physician usually makes rounds in the hospital may enable you to plan your visits to include that time.

Another source of information about your parent is a roommate. Roommates usually hear what is said to the other patient in the room. Roommates also know whether or not your parent went to x-ray, and may know how well your parent is eating. If your parent is in a private room, you will have to depend on your parent and the nursing staff for information.

Earlier in this chapter, I discussed establishing a relationship with your parent's physician. This process of clarifying your expectations may need to be repeated if consultants are called in to see your parent. With each new physician you need to establish a mutual understanding regarding information sharing and decision-making. Do not depend on the primary physician to pass along this information to consultants.

RESTRAINTS

A prime concern, and a legal responsibility, of the nursing staff is the safety of your parents (e.g., avoiding falls). Restraining your parent is one way to accomplish this. Restraints commonly used in hospitals are limb restraints and body restraints. Limb restraints are cloth bands, most commonly used on the wrist to prevent the patient from pulling out tubes such as nasogastric tubes or intravenous tubing. Body restraints are larger cloth bands placed across the upper part of the body, which may be used if there is a danger that the person would try to leave the bed and fall. Siderails are another "safety" device. Many hospitals have a policy that siderails must be raised on all patients who are sedated or over a certain age. Someone awakening in the middle of the night in a strange place and finding the way out of bed blocked by a siderail may attempt to climb over the siderail. This increases the likelihood that the person will fall and sustain an injury. Providing a nightlight for elderly patients is helpful.

There is a tendency to assume that most older people become confused in the hospital. The nurses, therefore, often restrain elderly people. A person who is accustomed to being "independent" may be humiliated. You may find it very difficult to see your parent "tied" into bed. You can always ask the reason for restraint. Remember, you are your parent's advocate. Perhaps you could work out an agreement with the nursing staff, if it seems appropriate based on your parent's condition, to have the restraints removed during your visit. It would then be your responsibility to notify staff when you are ready to leave.

REPLACING YOUR PARENT'S PHYSICIAN

It is possible that you may become dissatisfied with your parent's attending physician during your parent's stay in the hospital. If the problem is serious and cannot be resolved by discussion with the physician, you may wish to replace that physician. Replacement is possible while your parent is still in the hospital, but there are some protocols to follow. Your parent was admitted to the hospital by a particular physician and that physician is responsible for medical care while your parent is in the hospital. Usually only physicians are permitted to admit patients to the hospital. If you dismiss the admitting physician from the case, you must have a replacement. It is best to have the replacement lined up before you tell the admitting physician you do not wish him/her to see your parent any longer. Your parent should be involved in the decision about changing physicians.

Dissatisfaction with one physician may also be effectively handled by requesting consultation. You may be uneasy about the course your parent's illness or injury is taking. You may have some reservations about the admitting physician's skills in the area that seems to be the problem. It is your and/or your parent's right to request consultation. Some physicians react negatively to such a request. They interpret a request for consultation as an insinuation that they have not been doing their job well. This may be exactly your perception. It is not uncommon for physicians to lack skills or knowledge needed to care for elderly people. At any rate, you can request consultation. You can also request a specific consultant, a physician you know personally or one recommended by friends or relatives.

CONSULTATION

For a variety of reasons, you or the physician may request that a specialist see your parent during hospitalization. Following are some of the specialists you may encounter:

> Gastroenterologist—stomach, intestines, and related organs such as the liver, gall bladder
> Neurologist—diseases/conditions of the nervous system
> Neurosurgeon—surgery involving structures of the nervous system (brain, spinal cord, nerves)
> Oncologist—malignant diseases (cancer)
> Opthalmologist—disorders of the eyes
> Radiologist—interprets x-rays; administers radiation therapy
> Urologist—urinary tract
> Nephrologist—kidneys
> Cardiovascular specialist—heart and circulatory system
> Pulmonary specialist—lungs
> Psychiatrist, psychologist, psychiatric social worker—mental health

VISITORS

Often people think that elderly people are lonely and have few visitors. This may be the case when the elderly person is at home. Oddly enough, however, hospitalization sometimes stimulates "visiting." Your parent may be overwhelmed with visitors and become exhausted from trying to socialize with them. People respond differently to visitors. An elderly person who is weak from illness and/or diagnostic tests may prefer to see only close family. Other elderly people may welcome visitors and be pleased by the attention. Your parent should be involved in any decision to limit visitors.

If you and your parent decide it would be best to limit visitors, there are several courses of action you might try. One possibility is to suggest that people postpone their visits until your parent returns home and has regained strength. You can also ask the physician to restrict visitors and relay this "order" to persons you think might visit. It is best to head off visitors before they reach the hospital. Once visitors are in the hospital, it is difficult to refuse them "just a few minutes" with your parent. The hospital staff can stop only visitors who inquire about your parent or ask directions to your parent's room. People tend to think that a "No Visitors" sign refers to "other" visitors.

CAREGIVER AS VISITOR

Whether or not it is desirable for your parent to have other visitors, you, as caregiver, will want to visit as regularly as possible. If you find that you cannot visit as often as you want, or as often as you feel needed, perhaps a family member or close family friend could share the advocate role with you. Meal time is often a good time to visit, particularly if your parent needs help with eating. Many elderly people who are perfectly capable of feeding themselves sitting at a table at home may not be able to manage while in bed in a half sitting position. The nursing staff are usually rushed at meal time trying to feed a number of patients plus find time for their own meal breaks. In addition to providing companionship during a meal, you can encourage and assist your parent to eat at a more leisurely pace. Nurses sometimes feed patients very rapidly. Your parent may choose not to eat rather than "delay" a busy nurse.

Mental Status

While visiting your parent, it is important to note any change in behavior, particularly any changes in mental status. Common causes of confusion include infection, medication, or depression. Family members are in a much better position than the hospital staff to pick up confusion in the very early stages. If what your parent says seems unusual to you, call this to the attention of the nurse and/or the physician. Talking about someone who is dead as though they were alive is an example of confusion. Not remembering where they were living immediately prior to hospitalization is another example of confusion which may be obvious to you but not to the staff.

Emotional Support

One of the most important roles a family member can play for a hospitalized parent is to provide emotional support. If you have been providing physical care, this may be an opportunity for you to obtain some rest from this particular chore. However, your parent will continue to need your emotional support even more than when at home. Hospitals can be strange and frightening places, particularly to someone who is no longer able to negotiate an unfamiliar environment due to various physiological changes. Just being there—touching, talking, a familiar face and voice in unfamiliar surroundings—is important. Someone to explain and interpret can make the strangeness less frightening.

You may also want to provide some comfort measures for your parent. Just sitting can be frustrating for a caregiver, particularly when you see that your parent is not comfortable. In the hospital the primary responsibility for the nursing care of your parent rests with the nursing staff. There are things you can do for your parent that will add to his/her comfort. These include "forcing fluids," "mouth care," "foot massage," and "positioning."

Fluids

It is important to ask the nurse what kinds of fluids your parent is permitted and whether or not the amount is limited. Fluids are sometimes limited, for example, in certain cardiac conditions such as severe congestive heart failure, or they may be restricted because of tests or procedures.

If your parent is permitted fluids, it is desirable to maintain an adequate intake by mouth if at all possible. For a variety of reasons, many older people do not drink enough fluids. When you are visiting, it would be helpful if you encourage your parent to take fluids. It is easier to drink a small amount of liquid at frequent intervals instead of a large amount at one time. You are in a position to offer fluids more frequently than the nursing staff, and your parent's intake would be increased by having you (and other visitors) do so. Fluids other than water are usually available on request. These include coffee, tea, clear broth, and juices.

Mouth Care

A frequent complaint of hospitalized people is dry mouth. This may be due to a number of factors including effects of medication and fluid restrictions. Your parent may not complain of a dry mouth and may even deny having a dry mouth. It is still desirable to keep lips and mucous membranes moist. This can be done in a variety of ways. Sometimes a person who is not permitted fluids may have an occasional chip of ice which can dissolve in the mouth and alleviate the dryness. Many hospitals provide swabs that can be used to sponge out the inside of the mouth. One type of swab is a small, square sponge on a stick which can be dipped in water or a dilute mouthwash solution. The sponge doesn't taste particularly pleasant (to me) with plain water, but this is a matter of personal preference. There are also commercial products that provide "artificial" saliva. Some people find these sprays very helpful, while others do not like them. You can ask the nurse caring for your parent, or the physician, to order one of these products, or you can buy it yourself at a drugstore. Another frequently used measure to relieve dryness of the mouth is a glycerin and lemon swab. The glycerin provides lubrication but the lemon tends to be drying. These are more suitable for the interior of the mouth than the lips. A chapstick can be ordered from the pharmacy to keep lips lubricated. If your mother is accustomed to using cold cream on her lips, by all means encourage her to do so in the hospital and see that she has the cream. Plain glycerin is an excellent means of keeping the lips moist. Unfortunately it tastes awful!

FOOT MASSAGE—BENEFITS AND PRECAUTIONS

Foot massage is a comfort measure that is often overlooked, particularly in the hospital. A foot massage helps many people relax and may be particularly beneficial at bedtime. There are, however, times when a person's feet should not be massaged.

Do not massage your parent's feet without specific approval from the physician, if your parent has any of the following:

  a) skin lesions on the feet (e.g. cuts, or sores)
  b) fractures of the hip or any part of the leg
  c) phlebitis or thrombophlebitis (even if this is only suspected)
  d) severe arthritis pain in the feet

If your parent does not have any of the above problems, he/she may enjoy a foot massage.

First wash and dry the feet. If possible, soak the feet for ten minutes in warm water. Wash your hands with warm water—cold hands do not promote relaxation. Rub lotion or baby oil between the palms of your hands. Gently grasp one foot and hold it with both hands for a minute or two. This usually prevents initial ticklishness or jumpiness. Continue holding the foot in both hands and make circles with your thumbs over the entire sole of the foot. Next spread the sole with your fingers to relax tight muscles. Support the foot with one hand and stroke the sole with the knuckles of the other hand, using an up and down motion. Gently rotate each toe (unless your parent finds this uncomfortable). Lift the foot off the bed and knead the heel and ankle between your thumb and forefinger (or rub with fingertips). You will need to use a little more pressure when massaging the heel because the skin is thicker and coarser. Repeat the procedure with the other foot. (The source for much of the material on foot massage is: G. Joachim, "How to Give a Great Foot Massage," *Geriatric Nursing* [Jan./Feb. 1983]:28–29).

POSITIONING

If your parent cannot change position at will, you can often assist with positioning. Proper positioning and frequent changes of position can help to ease pain and lessen skin irritation or breathing problems. Sometimes just raising or lowering the head of the bed a couple of inches can make your parent more comfortable. Raising the knees may be helpful, but you will want to make sure there are no reasons not to do this. Pillows under the arms can help reduce the strain on shoulders or the upper part of the body. Pillows under the knees should be used with caution, however, as they may interfere with circulation to the lower part of the legs.

Helping your parent find comfortable positions while in bed can be a cooperative effort for you and the nursing staff. You may know from experience at home what positions your parent finds comfortable (or uncomfortable), especially for sleeping. The nurse may be able to demonstrate ways of moving and positioning your parent that will minimize the strain for you and the discomfort to your parent. Your ability to help the nurse reposition your parent will increase the likelihood that your parent's position will be changed often (every two hours is usually desirable).

DISCHARGE PLANNING

With the implementation of federal regulations governing length of stay (DRG's), a trend was noted toward discharging patients "quicker and sicker." This means that your parent may be discharged from the hospital before you believe he/she is ready to leave the hospital. You need to keep in mind when thinking about where your parent should go following hospitalization, that your parent may not be functioning as well as before hospitalization. Whatever the reason for the hospitalization, your parent is likely to experience some loss of functional abilities. Whether or not there will be a return to the level of functioning prior to hospitalization may not be readily apparent at this point. What this means is that even though you may have been caring for your parent at home before hospitalization, you may not be able to do so immediately following hospitalization.

Planning for your parent's eventual discharge from the hospital should begin immediately after admission. If at all possible, your parent should be involved in the planning and decision-making. In some hospitals the social worker is the person responsible for assisting you in planning for your parent's care after discharge. The team will usually include the social worker, the nurse who is most knowledgeable about your parent, and other appropriate health care professionals. It is desirable for you to have an active role in this process.

If your parent's discharge plan includes a period of convalescence in a nursing home, then the discharge planning process will begin again with the staff in that facility. Mary Anne, uninformed about this process at the time of her mother's discharge from the nursing home asked, "Where would she go?" Nursing homes usually have social workers, or designated discharge planners, who are knowledgeable about community resources and can help you plan.

SUMMARY

In this chapter I have tried to provide you, the caregiver, with information that will help you "negotiate the system" when your parent is hospitalized. You are your parent's advocate.

An advocate must be prepared to be unpopular. Persons who question the status quo are sometimes labeled "trouble makers." Being "deviant" has its price. You may find yourself an unwelcome visitor, shunned by the nursing and medical staff. If you find that it is necessary to "make waves" to get the care you believe your parent needs, by all means do so. You will sleep better.

REFERENCES AND SUGGESTED READINGS

American Association of Retired Persons (AARP) *A Handbook about Care in the Home.* Washington, DC: AARP, 1982
———. *Information on Medicare and Health Insurance for Older People.* Washington, DC: AARP, 1985.
———. *Medicare's Prospective Payment System: Knowing Your Rights.* Washington, DC: AARP, 1986.
———. *Your Home, Your Choice: A Workbook for Older People and Their Families.* Washington, DC: AARP, 1984.
Channing L. Bete Co., Inc. *About Medigap* (No. 1432 B-11-85). South Deerfield, MA: Channing L. Bete Co., 1985.
———. *How to Manage Your Medications* (No. 1432 D-2-86). South Deerfield, MA: Channing L. Bete Co., 1986.
———. *Physical Health in Later Years* (No. 1225 F-7-85). South Deerfield, MA: Channing L. Bete Co., 1986.
———. *Taking Care of Your Elderly Relatives* (No. 1296 B-7-85). South Deerfield, MA: Channing L. Bete Co., 1986.
———. *What Everyone Should Know about Skilled Nursing Homes* (No. 1169 C5-78). South Deerfield, MA: Channing L. Bete Co., 1982.
Health Care Financing Administration. *Guide to Health Insurance for People with Medicare* (No. 1979-296-540). Washington, DC: U.S. Government Printing Office, 1979.
———. *How to Select a Nursing Home* (DHHE Publication No. 1985-0-470-477). Washington, DC: U.S. Government Printing Office, 1980.
———. *Prospective Payment for Hospitals Under Medicare* (No. 1983-0-418-728 QL3). Washington, DC: U.S. Government Printing Office, 1983.
National Institute on Drug Abuse. *Using Your Medications Wisely: A Guide for the Elderly.* Washington, DC: AARP.
Peterson, J. *On Being Alone.* Washington DC: AARP, 1980.
Skolnick, B. *Prescription for Action: A Guide to Community Health Reform.* Washington, DC: AARP, 1984.

Skolnich, B., and R. Warrick. *The Right Place at the Right Time: A Guide to Long Term Care Choices*. Washington, DC: AARP, 1984.

Social Security Administration. *How to Complete the Patient's Request for Medicare Payment* (SSA Publication No. 05-10083). Washington, DC: U.S. Government Printing Office, 1983.

U.S. Consumer Product Safety Commission. *Home Safety Checklist for Older Consumers* (No. 1985-475-981: 32202). Washington, DC: U.S. Government Printing Office, 1985.

WHEN INDEPENDENCE IS NO LONGER POSSIBLE

A broken hip, a sudden illness, the death of a spouse, a decline because of chronic illness, the loss of memory . . . these are some of the points at which independence is threatened. It is at such points of crisis when families become even more closely involved as advocates and caregivers. In crisis then, facing strong feelings and new experiences, they find themselves trying to help with decisions regarding financial matters, acute health care, and long-term care.

Pat talks about her feelings, and the intricacies of the caregiving role when independence was no longer possible for her parents. "Feelings" by Dr. Barbara Silverstone was selected to be reprinted here for its helpful, informative approach to the wide range of feelings families experience. Linda, a nurse-attorney, discusses the complicated, confusing issue of decision-making in response to Pat, including such topics as autonomy, informed consent, refusing or withdrawing treatment, and surrogate decision-making.

My Parents Grew Old Right before My Eyes

Pat Meier

I began my story for this book at 3:25 A.M. on a July morning. It was a matter of deciding to turn a sleepless night into a more productive period by putting some of my inner turmoil on paper.

On the previous day I had observed my forty-sixth birthday—birthdays are always a time of reflective soul-searching for me. Part of the day had been spent with my parents, both residents of a nearby nursing home. I made sure I was my usual "cheerful" self, trying to make our visit pleasant, feeling that my parents' happiness depended on me—yet still being ill at ease after two years of such visits. (I don't believe I will ever quite get used to the idea of my parents residing in an institution rather than their home. Also I have the uneasy feeling that I am part of the reason for that situation, being physically and emotionally unable to care for my highly incapacitated mother and father in my home.) While I made preparations to serve the cake and ice cream I had brought, my mother commented that I would have to "feed the baby," referring to herself. Mother's severe arthritic condition has reduced her once capable hands to a state where she is virtually unable to feed herself, let alone perform personal services.

I began to feed Mother, taking occasional bites from my own plate, but scarcely tasting them. Meanwhile, I realized that I had erred in not placing my father's plate on the bed table rather than on his lap. But it was too late! I saw the plate, ice cream, and cake slide to the floor, and observed Daddy's embarrassment at having made a mess for me to clean up. I apologized for not having thought of the table, and quickly provided another plate for him. We chatted for a few minutes, and then my mother suggested that I return my father to his own room—in her opinion, he was probably tired. My father offered no resistance to her suggestion, so we said our polite thank you's and goodbyes—

Daddy had spoken no more than ten words during the entire visit. The systemic lupus erythematosus has begun to affect his facial muscles, making speech difficult.

I knew that my mother wanted our usual visit without Daddy, so after kissing my father and promising to return in a few days, I returned to her room. A favorite aide soon dropped in for cake, and then one of the activities people came by. My mother enjoyed the "girl talk," and it all helped to pass the time. It was a pleasant, sociable visit, yet underneath I felt annoyed and guilty because my mother had so firmly manipulated my father out of the picture.

I left the nursing home with a great sense of relief at being able to reenter the "real world." Nevertheless, the afternoon had gone fairly well, and I felt that I had fulfilled my obligation to my parents and myself by having had at least a semblance of a birthday celebration. It was then time to meet my husband, Bill, for the forty-five-minute drive to pick up our two sons at summer camp. Yesterday was the older one, Steve's, birthday also, and he had become a teenager! We stopped for an ice cream treat on the way home and caught up on the week's activities. This was a happier and more carefree time for me, as my thoughts of the visit to my parents were forgotten for now. But they were not really forgotten and were coming back this sleepless night as I reflected on the day's happenings and my forty-sixth birthday.

Ever since my parents have been residents in a nursing home, I have not looked forward to family birthdays and particularly not to Mother's and Father's Days—these holidays only emphasize how much I long for the old days when my parents were still able to be in their own home. That day the guilt feelings were very strong—they are always with me, I think, but I try to block them out most of the time. With the very valuable help of a support group for daughters of the elderly, I have come a long way in coping with this situation. However, it has made a lasting impression on me and has touched my life and the lives of my family deeply. In times like these I "let go" and weep for all of us!

THE WELL-TRAVELED ROAD

As an only child (my older brother died in his teens), my involvement in the care of Mother and Daddy had been growing over the past several years. After they were both involved in an auto accident, I began to visit them on a more regular basis—weekly rather than every two or three weeks as before. These visits kept me informed about their condition and also offered support for them during a very stressful time. Mother's condition was such that Daddy had become the caregiver. With the assistance of Meals-on-Wheels, Visiting Nurse, good neighbors (one of whom was an R.N.), and my weekly visits, he was able to care for my mother. He learned to change the bandages on her injured foot, clean the infected area, and rebandage—this had to be done several times each day.

Caring for my mother was in itself a stressful situation for my father. Their marriage of over fifty years had been a troubled one, and my mother's domineering attitude soon began to wear on his nerves. Hence, my weekly visits quickly became my entry into the "battle zone." Each parent would tell me that the other didn't understand. Unfortunately, this was nothing new for me as my parents had always competed for my attention, sympathy, and support. This position of being caught between them had always been very painful and frustrating for me but had never been resolved. Now it was especially distressing to leave my own family responsibility each week, make the one hundred-mile round trip, listen to an account of their problems, and try to make "peace."

Time spent on the road was approximately two and one-half hours, and visits usually lasted about three hours. As I drove to my parents' home, I was always wondering what would confront me *this* time, and on the trip back (usually in a hurry to pick up our youngest son at school) I spent the time going over what I had just experienced.

On trip days then, I was always extremely tired as well as physically and emotionally drained, so that the evening was never very pleasant for my husband and the boys. I hated to be so "down," but it was breaking my heart to watch my parents become so frail and not be able to do anything about it. Many times after I left their home, I spent part of the return trip crying and then giving myself a "pep talk"—sometimes I thought I must be losing my mind as my emotions flip-flopped! Although my husband had always been supportive, I began to feel guilty talking to him so much about my parents and their seemingly insoluable problems. Bill always asked how the visit had gone, but I felt sure he had to be tired of hearing the same news week after week. He had long ago realized that my parents manipulated me, but had been patient in not making a point of telling me. I believe he realized that I knew this was the situation but was unable to get myself out of the "little girl" trap.

Finally, one hot summer day, my mother and I had our first confrontation ever, and at the time I was forty-two years old! I am not certain exactly what triggered this outburst, but I know now that it was simply the accumulation of years of "holding back" on my part, and I finally exploded. I was not very proud of myself afterward, for I had never been permitted to talk back to my parents. Strangely enough, this episode was not followed by tremendous guilt as I expected but rather by a sense of relief. I am certain that my mother was hurt by my outburst, and of course, astonished. We never spoke of the incident again, but Mother was quite cool toward me for several weeks. However, she did not exert the same pressures on me for some time, so I felt I had accomplished something; I did regret that it took so many years to finally stand up for myself. My mother and I had always shared a very close relationship, and I realize now that as I grew up I never wanted to hurt or disappoint her. This, of course, is a totally unrealistic attitude to have in any relationship.

THE MOVE

My mother's arthritic condition had become complicated by a series of abcesses on her leg; these resulted in a staph infection which eventually led to her being hospitalized for eight weeks in isolation. About a year later my father entered the hospital for what I presumed to be mostly fatigue and, of course, the stress a caregiver normally encounters. Tests determined that my father had systemic lupus erythematosus which could be controlled with medication. Since his hospitalization, my mother had hired a live-in housekeeper. Although this was somewhat difficult for all involved, it seemed to work, but my parents felt they were losing their independence and their privacy. There was a series of housekeepers, some of them very competent, others impossible and irresponsible. I continued to make weekly trips to my parents' home (more often if one was hospitalized). Within one year, my father was hospitalized three times with lupus, and after one of these periods it was necessary for him to enter a nursing home. He remained in the nursing home for approximately two months and began learning to walk again. He was looking forward to going home; in fact, this goal provided an incentive to his therapy. Unfortunately, during the next year he suffered a total collapse. The current housekeeper was very capable but had back problems and stated that she could not lift both my father and mother. Therefore, she would be forced to quit caring for my parents. Realizing that their health problems required more than one person could do for them, my parents now began to talk about moving to a nursing home together. "Talk" was all they did until my father was hospitalized once again—this time with severe depression and neutropenia (a blood disorder) in addition to the pre-existing condition. Now my husband and I made the suggestion that they enter a nursing home near us and sell their home. With their consent, I selected a nursing home and started the paperwork. My father left the hospital fifty miles away and was brought by ambulance to a nursing home approximately twenty minutes from our home. Within two days my mother was also admitted. She also traveled by ambulance, as she had developed a very painful back condition, no doubt due in part to the severe stress she was undergoing. I realize now that leaving her home was much more traumatic for Mother than she revealed. As a "cover up" for her sadness, her last days in the house were filled with frantic preparations for the move. She told me that she had taken care of everything; I was free of any responsibility. Mother, unfortunately, was on the brink of collapse—physically and emotionally. Bill and I visited Mother and Daddy at the nursing home every day that first week; then Mother asked that we not feel that we had to come so often. In the meantime, my parents' furniture was moved and stored near us. The color TV, writing desk, and a favorite chair were to be moved into my mother's room but my father made no requests for personal items. My parents chose to live in separate rooms. In view of their troubled marriage and diminished physical condition they would feel much more comfortable not being together twenty-four hours a day. This arrangement, incidentally, has worked out very well for them in spite of some raised eyebrows from outsiders. This was their decision and I wanted to honor their wishes.

MOVING DAY

On the day Mother and Daddy's furniture and personal belongings were to be moved and stored near us, I arrived at their home shortly before the movers. I had taken the boys with me for company on the trip, but more importantly for their support during the move. My parents were now residents of the nursing home, and once the furniture and contents were moved, their former home and mine would be just another "house for sale."

The movers arrived and began their work. The packed boxes and furniture, representing a family's lifetime, were loaded on a moving van in about two and one-half hours. I felt that day, and for several days afterward, that my parents had died and that I was merely "cleaning up."

While the men were working, a neighbor I had previously met stopped by to ask me about buying some of the articles. She did not inquire about my parents health or their new location or even bother to engage in small talk. I was furious at her insensitivity but held my Irish temper until she had left the house. Steve, then eleven, said, "Why were you so rude to that lady?" "She was no lady, but a ghoul," I sputtered. This statement was perhaps a little dramatic but those were my feelings at the time. I had been told earlier in the day by one of the workers that I should have had an auction and saved the expense of the move!

Other neighbors, friends of my parents, stopped in for a few last words. I appreciated their interest, and I knew how difficult it was for them to lose their long-time neighbors. One woman mentioned how much she would miss seeing the lights come on in the evening at my parents' home.

The workers finished; I checked the house once more for any forgotten items and locked the front door. I was crying as we drove away, but the mood was broken when Eric, our eight-year-old, reminded me that it was time for lunch. The boys never forget mealtime and today was no exception! I was glad to have them with me.

When we arrived at the building where my parents' furniture and personal belongings were to be stored, I asked one of the workers if he had delivered Mother's special requests to her room at the nursing home. He said that he had, but when I asked if Mother had any comments he said, "Lady, I didn't talk to her. I didn't want to spend any more time than I had to in that place." I have never been able to hide my feelings very well and this was certainly one of those times. He seemed embarrassed after his thoughtless statement and our conversation ended.

The move had been completed. My parents were in their new home, and I felt a sense of relief. The new living arrangements would not be perfect, but at least Mother and Daddy were just twenty minutes away now.

My parents rarely mention their former home, but just last spring Daddy was wondering if the new residents were enjoying the spring bulbs he loved so much. I have no desire to see the house again—it is still too painful for me. That chapter of my life and my parents' is closed forever.

ADJUSTMENT PROBLEMS

Adjustment to living in a nursing home has to be one of life's "downers." My father never said much other than to complain about the food and all the "nuts" running around. My mother was too cheerful and too satisfied—I should have known there were problems. Within three months, she became "different"— sometimes confused, sometimes depressed. Within another two months she lapsed into a severe depression and needed psychiatric treatment. Fortunately, the psychiatrist who cared for her was very interested in and had many geriatric patients. My mother's basic problem was that she had play-acted her way through life, appearing to be what she thought people wanted her to be and covering up all her hurts and disappointments. After revealing these to the psychiatrist and working through them, she was like a new person—the mother I had not had in years. It was a happy time for us as we had always been close and shared, among other things, a rather zany sense of humor. Once again Mother was interested in other people and not just in her own problems. Unfortunately, her health problems continued, and each illness pulled her down while recovery seemed to take twice as long as it had in past years.

One of these illnesses occurred when Mother became toxic from medication and developed a psychotic depression. She was hospitalized for one week, and it was sheer horror for her and all concerned. A friend's mother had been toxic from medication three times, and each time I heard the terrible stories I thought I knew how bad the situation really was. Until my own mother became toxic, I did not really understand how frightening an experience it would be for all of us. She was in constant pain; real or imagined, it did not matter because the cries of anguish that I heard tore me apart. Yet I was unable to do anything about it. Although my mother appeared to recognize me and everyone who visited, she drifted in and out, suffering her pain and despair and feeling, I am certain, abandoned by all. For the first time, she had to be restrained to prevent her from pulling out the feeding tube that was helping her to survive this ordeal. My mother is still very frail, now up to about eighty pounds. One of the blessings has been that she remembers very little of those several weeks when she was certainly not herself.

I was eager to have my mother return to the nursing home, as I felt that she would receive better care there than in the hospital, inasmuch as there was no geriatric unit, and the personnel were not sufficiently trained in caring for the special needs of the frail elderly. In fact, the morning after my mother was admitted to the hospital a nurse told me to keep her quiet or she would have to be moved to a private room. I was so exhausted from the night before that I let this pass, but I did tell the doctor that I thought it was one of the most insensitive remarks that could have been made under the circumstances. I assumed, correctly, that the nurse would be reprimanded, and the next day when I saw her again, her attitude had changed to one of concern.

While Mother was hospitalized, I continued to be a "pest" as far as the staff was concerned, but whatever it took for my mother to receive adequate care, I did. Fellow support group members stayed with Mother so that my husband, children, and I could get away for an already-planned weekend during this time. As I look back, Mother's episode with drug toxicity was a nightmare, and due to the circumstances of Mother's toxic condition, I have continued to monitor her medication given at the nursing home. If the doctor changes the medication or dosage, I want to know about it.

GUILT

It became obvious to me one evening that my family had no ideaof my feelings of fear and frustration. I was having difficulty establishing a balance between concerns about long-term care for my parents and the daily demands of my family. That evening a poster that our support group had taken to the NCOA (National Council on Aging) National Conference was still in my family room. The poster portrayed a woman being pulled by her husband and children on one side, with her parent in a wheelchair on the other side, plus a small dog tugging at the hem of her dress. Steve asked, "Mom, is that the way your really feel?" This incisive query came from the same son who had some weeks earlier complained that "the family could starve," because I had not done my weekly grocery shopping but had worked several hours in the support group office.

I do want to emphasize that my husband and children have been supportive and helpful in their individual ways in the care of my parents. Additionally, members of the support group have for three years seen me through many crises, including some of which my family was not aware. I remember very clearly now, how for at least two years prior to finding the group, I kept searching for someone who would be understanding of my situation with my parents, someone I could talk to without sounding like a whining complainer. When I discovered the support group quite by chance, I was happy to have others who shared similar problems. That very special bonding has remained a most important factor in my association with the other daughters. These women care; they are nonjudgmental and want to help in any way possible.

One issue I have been dealing with for three years is guilt. This feeling may not seem "logical" to outsiders since it appears that the child is doing whatever needs to be done for the parents. If this means specialized care in a nursing home, why should one continue to feel guilty?

Madeleine L'Engle, in her book, *The Summer of the Great-Grandmother*,[1] discusses the difference between real guilt and false guilt. If we can examine our guilt feelings, realize that some are real, and then assume responsibility for our actions or admit our errors, real guilt becomes a release for us—finished business. In contrast, false guilt never gives us a feeling of being released and is a source of stress and fatigue. I visit my parents every week, but I'm always in a rush, always running. I could easily fall into the trap of guilt by wondering if my weekly visits are enough, even though I know how supportive these visits have been to my parents. The real trap is "false guilt" when I berate myself for not being able to care for them in my home. Nevertheless, it is very difficult for me to be logical where Mother and Daddy are concerned. I find it very frustrating to discuss this subject with my husband. He is so detached and logical, while I am so emotionally involved! No one knows in advance how they would react if placed in such a position—logic might fly out the window!

INNER FEELINGS

Many articles have been written on the feelings associated with the death of a loved one: shock, denial, anger, depression, and finally acceptance. I believe that children of frail, elderly parents experience these same feelings. Another feeling I have experienced often is frustration at my inability to prevent the chain of events that, I know, will lead to the eventual loss of my parents. Frustration can lead to stress, and in the case of children of frail elders, it can be devastating unless we are able to come to terms with it. I have been very depressed as the health of my parents has steadily deteriorated, and I have been helpless to prevent it. Helpless—unable to help oneself; incapable; inefficient; these are a few definitions from the dictionary. I believe it is also the loss of control of a situation. In past months, my feelings of helplessness have led to a great deal of stress resulting in migraine and tension headaches, digestive disorders, and a hair-trigger temper. I realize that I must find ways to reduce my stress level so that I can function in a more healthful manner. After all, if I am ill I can be of help to no one, including my husband, children, and parents.

Each of us must find outlets to reduce the stress in our lives. I know that when I exercise I feel better and more able to cope with my problems; I also find music to be a stress reducer. Of course, being able to talk with others who are in similar circumstances is of tremendous help, but there are many times when you must deal with your problems alone; then you must have some resources available to use as coping skills. One way to begin is by allowing yourself time for an activity that is relaxing and meaningful for you. As caregivers, we must remember to nurture ourselves and leave the guilt feelings behind—where they belong.

WHERE DO YOUR PARENTS LIVE?

This is a simple enough question, but one I have found increasingly difficult to answer ever since my parents became residents of a nursing home. Upon hearing the answer, it seems to me that most people respond with shock and embarrassment. There seems to be no graceful way out for either of us once this question has been posed. The words "nursing home" have had such unpleasant connotations for so many years that I feel immediate guilt for having placed my parents in such a situation. "What is the state of their health?" is usually the next question plus the unstated belief that it could be possible for *both* to be in this type of facility. After a brief explanation of the health problems involved, the subject is closed, much to the relief of the inquirer and myself. Logically, I know there was no choice, and fortunately, my parents have been very cooperative and understanding in this delicate matter. Yet living with this decision has been painful. Occasionally, I still wonder if I could have cared for my parents in my home, with my husband, a teenage son, and a preteen son. However, after each visit to our home by my parents, I know there is no way we could care for even one parent, let alone two. As our group facilitator, a registered nurse, has reminded me—more than once—my parents require nursing care. As for learning to accept the decision and visiting my parents in the nursing care facility, there will always be some doubt in my mind.

I have learned that there are times when we have few choices available. I feel strongly that the general public must be educated regarding the care of the frail elderly. We never know how our parents' health will change from day to day, so it is not always possible to plan pleasant transitions. With better education about health care facilities, respite for caregivers, and a general awareness of the study of geriatrics, we can insure better care not only for our parents but also for ourselves. Our children will be facing many of the same problems we are facing now—let's give them something better than the sometimes "hit-or-miss" information we have been given. Let us also hope that our children will be able to answer the question "Where do your parents live?" without experiencing as much emotional turmoil as many of us do at present.

WHAT ABOUT LIFE SUPPORTS?

The question of life supports is a crucial subject that I must discuss with my parents. What kinds of life supports are acceptable? What is the difference between life supports and supportive care? As I mentioned earlier, my mother was critically ill several months ago as a result of drug toxicity. Although I knew Mother had been depressed, I was stunned by the rapid deterioration of her mental condition. My parents were at our home for a Mother's Day dinner, and my mother's behavior was bizarre. She believed my father, who was seated near her at the dining table, was dead and had been replaced by a lifelike robot. Although she had refused to eat for several days and her weight was approximately eighty pounds, her daily medication dosages had not been reduced, allowing the toxic condition to develop—she was being poisoned!

On the Wednesday following Mother's Day we were notified that Mother's condition was serious. Then at midnight, Mother's nurse called to tell us she was about to be taken by ambulance to the hospital emergency room. Bill and I quickly dressed and told the children we had to leave. We arrived at the hospital ahead of the ambulance.

When Mother arrived at the hospital, she appeared to recognize us but was in great pain from violent muscle spasms. The spasms began at her head and continued along the length of her body, causing her stiffened limbs to jerk painfully and uncontrollably. After what seemed an eternity her psychiatrist telephoned and ordered intravenous medication to relieve the spasms. This treatment was successful, and she was finally able to rest. The next few days were critical—Mother's will to live had vanished. Her world was unreal for the most part, and she begged God to let her die. Within a few days the accumulated poisons began to leave her body, but she could not chew or swallow solid food. As she was in need of nourishment, her psychiatrist suggested tube feedings. I agreed to this as I knew she needed to build up her strength if she was to recover. Another physician on the case telephoned to tell me that he did not agree with the use of tube feedings and would prefer to be released from responsibility for Mother if the tube feedings were initiated. His remarks seemed to imply that due to Mother's age (seventy-four) and frailty, there was not much he felt could be done for her. I sought advice from the group facilitator and later from the group. As we discussed concerns about the problem, I realized that the "right" answer or approach may differ from situation to situation. We reached the conclusion as we talked that Mother was certainly entitled to food in this case as her illness was acute, and that the administering of food would not be a means of prolonging life as much as a chance to let the body regain some strength. The group supported my decision to proceed with the tube feedings. The outcome was a happy one—Mother did regain her strength and her will to live. Later she observed that she was glad to be alive and to celebrate her seventy-fifth birthday. However, should this situation arise again, I want to have a knowledge of my parents' thoughts on this subject. How very difficult it is to be responsible for determining how and when a person's life shall end, especially when that person is your parent.

PREPARING FOR THE LOSS OF PARENTS

I have given more thought in recent months to the time when I must give up my parents. Of course this is inevitable, but since both are so frail, I think about death more often. When I think about my parents I am usually concerned for their well-being, state of mind, and comfort.

Anticipating the loss of my parents, I think back to several instances in the past few years when I was certain that they would not recover. Each time I prepared myself for that loss and was so relieved when death did not occur. Now, I have almost reached the point where I cannot bear to think of their having to suffer once again, and part of me prays for a peaceful death for them.

We are always our parents' children, even though we spend years trying to prove we are adults. Even when we marry and rear a family of our own, it is somehow comforting to know that we are someone's child. When we lose our parents, we are no longer someone's daughter—a title that can never be ours again. I had never really thought about the significance of this until one of the daughters lost her mother and, in her grief, shared this recognition.

AFTER MOTHER'S DEATH

Three years have passed since most of my story was written, and I find in re-reading it that some of the memories are still very painful to me. My mother's death and my father's rapidly deteriorating health since that time have added another dimension to my life. Although I thought I was prepared for my mother's death, I learned after the initial shock and "acceptance" of my loss that my grieving did not diminish but seemed to intensify. We are not allowed enough time by our society to properly grieve for our loved ones. Usually, most of our grieving is done in the privacy of our homes as we are not encouraged to talk about our loss in public—it is too depressing a subject for discussion. Dr. Glen W. Davidson in his book, *Understanding Mourning*,[2] gives us no time limit. What a relief it was to read his book and learn that I am "normal" in spite of my crying jags, depression, dreams of the deceased, and so on. In the year that has passed since my mother's death I have observed holidays, family birthdays, and anniversaries without her—my "formal" mourning period has ended. Although I continue to miss her, I find that I am able to speak about her without as much sadness.

I had often heard the words "finality of death," but their meaning had never had the impact they now have for me. I was not prepared for the longing to be able to see Mother again. This feeling was quite a surprise, as her last months of life were spent in such pain, and because of dramatic weight loss, she didn't even look like herself. In the last few weeks of Mother's life I told her (I don't even know if she heard me, as she drifted in and out of consciousness) that I was ready to give her up because I loved her too much to see her continue to suffer.

Now I face the loss of my father, whose health is very poor after a series of strokes. He is unable to speak and is, at times, so confused that any hope of settling unfinished business has been lost.

REMINISCING

Sometimes, as I sit with him, I think back to the days when I visited Mother here. Her severe health problems limited her participation in many of the nursing home activities, and our time together was usually spent in conversation. One afternoon I took a box of old family photographs to the nursing home for Mother to identify. These were very old photographs of relatives who died before I was born, and now their identity was known only to my mother. As we sifted through the box of photos, Mother made comments about the individuals and remembered happier times in her life. In more recent photos, we both noted the family resemblance between my deceased brother and me. Since Mother tired easily, the task of identifying the photos took several afternoons, and we were proud of our accomplishment. I believe this was an especially important experience for my mother as she felt useful, perhaps for the first time since entering the nursing home, and knew she was making an important contribution to the preservation of our family history. It was a fulfilling experience for me, as well, as the photos ceased to be just "family pictures" and became "real people." There were times during those months, though, that I hesitated to reminisce with Mother, since many times the pleasant memories seemed to trigger very painful ones for her as well.

I think back, too, to the days after my father entered the nursing home; he refused to talk with anyone, including me. My attempts at conversation resulted in one-word answers from Daddy. Later, it was quite a surprise to learn from our oldest son of his conversations with his grandfather in which my father spoke of his youth, growing up on a farm. His stories of borrowing his father's guns (without permission), skinny-dipping with his brothers in a nearby river (also without permission), and playing hookey from school made a frail grandfather become a "regular person" to his teenaged grandson.

Letting go of our parents is one of life's experiences that everyone must face. Daddy's condition now is difficult for me to accept, but I am happy to have my father and to know that he is able to recognize me and my family.

REFERENCES

1. Madeline L'Engle, *The Summer of the Great-Grandmother* (New York: Farrar, Straus & Giroux, 1974).
2. Glen W. Davidson, *Understanding Mourning* (Minneapolis: Augsburg, 1984).

RECOMMENDED READINGS

Bloomfield, Harold H., with Leonard Felder. *Making Peace with Your Parents*. New York: Random House, 1983.

Burger, Sarah Greene, and Martha D'Erasmo. *Living in a Nursing Home: A Complete Guide for Residents, Their Families and Friends*. New York: Seabury Press, 1976.

Halpern, Howard M. *Cutting Loose: A Guide to Adult Relationships with Your Parents*. New York: Simon & Schuster, 1977.

O'Connor, Nancy. *Letting Go with Love: The Grieving Process*. Apache Junction, AZ: Mariposa Press, 1984.

Silverstone, Barbara, and Helen Kandel Hyman. *You and Your Aging Parent: The Modern Family's Guide to Emotional, Physical, and Financial Problems*. Rev. and enl. ed. New York: Pantheon, 1982.

Feelings

Barbara Silverstone

There is a growing concern about how families feel about their aging parents—particularly on the part of that member who is providing a great deal of care to the older person. If she (and sometimes he) is feeling "good" about what she is doing, then presumably all is well and the daughter will continue in her caregiving tasks. If not, it is commonly assumed that the family caregiving will soon shift to another relative, to an agency or to a nursing home. However, nothing could be farther from the truth. Actually, daughters and sons lend a helping hand or provide a great deal of care to their parents regardless of how they feel and "give up" only under very pressing circumstances.

What *is* true is that a wide range of feelings characterize the relationship between the adult child and aging parent, though marked by differences between families and among members in any one family. Certainly, when more positive feelings prevail on both sides of the relationship, the caregiving task is easier. But even in the best of situations negative feelings can emerge. I shall describe some of the more common feelings families experience and suggest ways in which these feelings can be productively handled.

ON THE POSITIVE SIDE

Positive family feelings do abound and can range from intense affection and love between the generations to—simply—respect, concern and a responsible sense of "doing what is right." Yet some or all of these feelings may be present. Affection and love, for example, may not accompany other positive feelings. Growing out of a history of relationships that often defy understanding, these warm feelings cannot be turned off and on like a water spigot. Present as well as past behavior of the aging parent can have a strong impact. The elder who is able to maintain a strong investment in the younger generation and has sufficient energy to socialize will, understandably, elicit more affection from his children than the older person who is self-involved and non-giving.

Satisfaction is a positive feeling often experienced by adult children who care for aging parents. Not infrequently, adult children, if asked, will agree that it is rewarding to reciprocate the love and care given to them by their parents in earlier years. When the whole family shares this reciprocity, they may discover a "togetherness" never before experienced.

The reciprocal relationships between adult children and their adult parents has, unfortunately, been dubbed by some as a form of role reversal, particularly if the older person is very dependent on his or her children. This notion, which suggests that the adult child has become like a parent and the aging parent like his or her child, is not only inaccurate but harmful to both generations. The heightened dependency and handicaps that sometimes accompany old age should not be confused with the behavior of a child. If aging parents are *regarded* as childlike, they can easily be *treated* as children, in turn, increasing their dependency and possibly undermining their self-esteem. Additionally, when adult children try to see themselves in the parent role, the emotional somersault involved can result in some of the negative feelings we shall discuss later. Rather, adult children should view themselves as *dependable* other adults on whom aging parents can rely to greater or lesser degrees. Their strong caring feelings emanate from the earlier bond with the aging parent, but never replicate it.

ON THE NEGATIVE SIDE

While the positive aspects of caring for aging parents are strongly associated with loving and satisfying feelings, there are decidedly negative features which can engender anxiety, worry, resentment, anger and guilt on the part of adult children. These feelings may be self-inflicted or directed toward the aging parent or other family members. They may be related to the burdens of caregiving; to family conflict, past or present, stirred up by the older person's condition or need; and, perhaps most strongly, to the losses being experienced by the older person and his or her family members and the disequilibrium caused to the family as a whole.

The burdens of caregiving are directly related to the condition of the older person. Those suffering mental impairment—such as that caused by Alzheimer's disease—create the greatest burden for family caregivers, and among these sufferers the most difficult to care for are the incontinent and those with behavioral difficulties. The encroachments on the time and energy, particularly when the cargiving task stretches out over months and years, understandably create resentment, perhaps anger toward the older person, and the ensuing guilt over having such unacceptable feelings toward a frail, weak person—particularly one's own mother or father.

This situation takes on more significant proportions when one family member provides most of the care to the aging parent. Referred to as the primary caregiver, this person is most often, next to the older wife, an adult daughter. This pattern of family is preferred by many older persons who, in their heightened dependency, may need a strong bond with a close relative. It may also be an accident of geography, a lack of siblings, or simply the choice of the adult daughter. Whatever the reason, the potential for heightened negative feelings is far greater than when the burden is shared.

In spite of the strong one-to-one relationship that seems to develop in the caring for an aging parent, the involvement of other family is inevitable. Sisters and brothers, cousins and grandchildren, and, of course, husbands and wives, all have relationships with the older person and play critical roles in socializing, planning, money mangement and respite. Just as the greater involvement with an elder may enhance family togetherness and warm feelings, it may also create or revive family friction.

Jealously of the primary caregiver and the bond she has with the aging parent can occur. Latent competition between adult siblings—long ago put aside—may emerge over such issues as "what is best for mother?" Resentment by the primary caregiver over his or her having to carry so much of the burden is not uncommon. The geographically distant, relatively uninvolved son and daughter who still curry an aging parent's favor is a familiar stimulant of sibling rivalry and resentment.

The older person's relationship with his or her children over the years can culminate in highly emotional situations when frailty strikes. A domineering parent, who over the years demanded much and gave little, may face an abundance of guilt and anger from children no longer afraid to be forthright with their pent-up feelings.

Strong, unpleasant feelings are also aroused by the aging parent's deteriorating condition and the losses already experienced or anticipated. Mourning, for some families, begins long before death, particularly in situations where mental impairment changes an elder's personality or severely affects his or her memory and ability to recognize loved ones. Sadness and fear for one's own aging are normal reactions.

The helplessness which adult children feel in the face of persistent deterioration and illness adds to an already full array of emotions. Although nothing can be done to provide greater comfort to an elder or to improve their condition, adult children often experience feelings of failure at not being able to fully repay their parents for all they did in the past. The guilt over this self-inflicted sense of failure and helplessness can be powerful and ongoing even after the death of the parent.

Finally, the feelings of discomfort and anxiety shared by all in the family when their life is disrupted deserve mention. The burdens of caregiving, worry about the elder, stirred up emotions from the past, and reawakened relationships, place stresses on the family as a whole. The family, immediate and distant, can be thrown into disarray, and a new balance must be sought—for better or worse.

A JUGGLING ACT

It is the "better or worse" which I would like to address: that balance of positive and negative feelings within one family member, particularly the primary caregiver; that between the adult child and the aging parent; and that among the family members as a whole. I have suggested so far that both sets of feelings, seemingly contradictory at times and unexpressed, are present in families faced with the stresses of an ill or handicapped older person who depends on them for c_. and support. How these feelings are handled may seem like a juggling act; but the quality of the balancing process is critical to the family's and elder's peace of mind.

For the individual family member, particularly the primary caregiver, there must be room in her life for expression of the variety of feelings she is experiencing. For some, just the knowledge that contradictory positive and negative feelings toward an aging relative or other family member are acceptable will suffice. But, for most of us, validation is required from others whom we trust. Perhaps most important to the adult child is a spouse or other confidant who can hear her out without judgment or fault. The emotional isolation of the caregiver is to be avoided at all costs.

An important source of validation that adult sons and daughters often overlook is the aging parent who is not severely mentally impaired. It is surprising to some how an elderly parent will respond to feelings of an adult child if they are expressed. The fear of upsetting a parent or overburdening them in their fragile state holds us back. For some, the thought of expressing a negative feeling to a parent appears forbidden.

What is overlooked in these situations is the undisputed fact that most aging parents, no matter how ill, querulous or depressed, are concerned about their sons and daughters and their physical as well as emotional well-being. They require clear and direct feedback such as a statement from an adult daughter that she is feeling irritated and overburdened and needs a little time by herself to recoup or that she is annoyed with her mother for the late night phone calls which interrupt her sleep. The guilt aging parents may already be feeling over being a burden to their children, rather than being increased, can be relieved by giving them an active role in responding to their son or daughter's situation and adjusting their behavior. Keeping in mind that hearing impairments and mild confusion are not uncommon to older persons, it is imperative that these communications be clearly stated and repeated. Of course, there are aging parents too ill, self-involved or mentally confused to respond appropriately. But in many situations it is worth a try.

Meeting with other caregivers caught in similar situations is a well-proven way of handling feelings. These so-called "self-help" groups have increased in popularity in many areas of the country, sponsored by churches, temples, social agencies and hospitals. Of particular note is the nationwide network of groups sponsored by the Alzheimer's Disease and Related Disorders Association for family members with relatives suffering from this severely impairing disease. Repeatedly, the common theme heard by participants is "I no longer feel so alone." The realization that others suffer the same burdens and harbor similar feelings is very supportive and places these feelings in a healthy perspective.

The family itself, in addition to the elder, is an important means of relieving the tension of pent-up hidden feelings, not only for the primary caregiver, but for all involved. At that time when relatives are brought together to plan for and with an aging parent in crises, feelings and emotions should not be overlooked.

A step aside here to mention family communication is important. Poor communication can be a source of bad feelings, only exasperating an already difficult situation. It is important that all family members affected by the crises of an aging relative in need of care be openly involved in the decision-making process. This, of course, also includes the older person if he or she is mentally able. Secret communications or omitting a critical member can only lead to misunderstandings and resentment. The relative who lives at a distance is not necessarily disinterested in the welfare of an aging parent, and, parenthetically, may have a great deal to contribute, such as money, visits and respite.

An important benefit in terms of feelings is that—if they can indeed be shared among family members without acrimonious exchanges about past issues that should have been resolved long ago—a new pattern of family coping can emerge in which the feelings related to the present crises can be shared and accepted for what they are. Emotional baggage from the past that obstructs productive communications among family members may require the help of a professional counselor.

Last, but not least, are the actions which can be taken to attack the source of bad feelings. We have already mentioned improving poor family communications. Planning carefully and seeking professional consultation and as much information and facts as possible can help to forestall the guilty confusion that ensues when we make precipitous decisions. Accepting our own human limits in a busy life with other priorities such as job, children, husband or wife and our own health is essential. Seeking respite from the day-to-day caregiving situation and gaining control over our lives is critical to a sense of well-being. Here, another relative, friend, home health aide or day program can supplement our efforts. Even nursing home placement may be needed. The burden of providing 24-hour-a-day care for a chronically impaired elder may simply be too much for the family's mental and physical health.

IN CLOSING

The powerful feelings and emotions that propel family life, undergirded by intergenerational responsibility, are called into play when the crises of caring for an aging parent face us. Love and affection can be intertwined in various degrees with resentment, worry, anxiety, sadness, and guilt and extend well beyond the caregiving relationship to the entire family. Active steps are required to relieve the emotional isolation and burdens of the primary caregiver and, if needed, improved family communications including those with the older person. What comes spontaneously for some families may have to be more consciously pursued by others—a small price to pay for relative peace of mind during one of the most stressful situations facing a family: caring for an aging parent.

Decision-Making in Health Care

Linda Moskowitz

The legal aspects of health care decision-making is a complex topic. Although it may not be immediately apparent to them, patients (and their families) are confronted with a whole series of decisions concerning treatment during the course of any illness. None of these questions are easy, and usually the family members are totally unprepared for the difficult task that befalls them. In the best of situations the health care providers (nurses, doctors, social workers) will be sensitive, thoughtful, and helpful to the patients and their families. However, in many instances, the family will be left to deal with the decisions alone and uninformed. The problems are compounded by the necessity for the family to make the choices in the midst of crisis, when they are grappling with the reality of an illness, impending death, hospitalization or institutionalization of a loved one. It is in the nature of the situation that these decisions are overwhelming. Often they involve tragic choices, with the family required to choose between two agonizing alternatives.

Confronting the questions before the crisis can ease the burden for the family in many ways. If the possible choices are discussed while the patient is mentally able to understand the alternatives and to make his own choices (competent), the family will not be forced into the role of surrogate (substitute) decision-maker without any hint of what the patient wants for himself. Many vehicles are available to the individual who wishes to direct his or her own health care choices. These potential directives are governed by state law, but in most states,

Linda D. Moskowitz, JD, RN, is a nurse-attorney practicing in Valparaiso, Indiana. She is the president of Legal Resources for Nursing, a consulting and educational services firm serving health care professionals. Ms. Moskowitz has published widely, taught in both nursing and law schools, and presented workshops nationwide.

include the possibilities of living wills, voluntary guardianships, and durable powers of attorney. In some states there are other legal arrangements possible. The specific documents usually require some assistance of an attorney or organization who has dealt with the particular legal requirements of that state.

The way in which the questions are presented, the information made available by the health care providers and others, the process to enable the decision-making to go on—each part of the decision-making process—is governed by legal concepts. The law, of course, is changing constantly. It reflects societal mores and ethics, both those of the health care professionals and those of the public at large. Furthermore, the law develops primarily on a state-by-state basis (what is the law in New Jersey is not necessarily the law in Califorina, for example). These two factors have created confusion regarding the legality of treatment decisions for health care providers. In turn, the patients and families affected directly are often uninformed, frustrated, and stymied, at best; or, in some instances, purposely misled and denied their basic right to make their own choices (often called the rights of autonomy and self-determination).

The protection of patient autonomy in the decision-making process is a major thrust of court decisions and legal thinking. The patient's right to decide is often mistakenly called the patient's right to die, but in fact it is much broader than that. The right to decide encompasses the right to consent, the right to refuse consent, and the right to choose between available alternative treatments.

Pat Meier's story illustrates the unique nature of each patient's situation and the way in which the autonomy issue may arise. When her mother was toxic from medications, Pat requested tube feedings for her mother at the suggestion of one physician. Another physician implied tube feedings were the wrong decision, and that due to her mother's age and frail condition, not much could be done for her. Because of her own personal strengths and insight and the opportunity to talk to the support group, Pat was apparently able to grapple with the issues and reach her own conclusion. She was not, however, provided that opportunity or encouraged in her deliberations by the attending physician. He indicated his intention to withdraw from the case if she went forward with the tube feedings. How many other family members would have had the fortitude and group support that was available to Pat? How many other family members would have had the knowledge or a friend who was a geriatric nurse? How many other family members would have been able to exercise their legal rights in this situation?

Pat's situation also graphically illustrates that the rights we are discussing are the rights to live, to choose, to be appropriately informed, as well as the perhaps more dramatic rights to die or to have treatment terminated. Court cases have understandably focused on terminal patients for whom the choice not to be treated was likely to result in death in a short time. Predictably, those situations have created the most conflicts between patients and their health care providers, who are interested in prolonging life and in providing treatment. However, most patient choice situations are not decided or established in courtrooms. Most situations need not pit the family against the doctor. Even those with inherent conflict are usually resolved without being forced into the courts for decision. The education of patients and their families serves a most important purpose in preventing treatment decisions from becoming the subject of court cases.

It is obvious that there are many philosophical, legal, and ethical considerations (perhaps we might say conflicts) that can be inherent in treatment decisions. These situations are common for doctors and nurses, but are uncommon for the others directly involved. That alone can compound the conflicts between the professionals and the patient's family. Questions confronted by seriously ill patients (to treat or not, to hospitalize or not, to resuscitate or not) are profoundly disturbing for both the families and the professionals to consider. The questions do not lead obviously to any easy answers nor to any ideal solutions. As medical technology makes it possible to live longer, patients and their families are increasingly asserting their rights to choose whether they will depend upon that medical technology.

The President's Commission on the Study of Ethical Problems in Medicine and Biomedical and Behavioral Research noted, "Once someone realizes that the time and manner of death are substantially under the control of medical science, he or she wants to be protected against decisions that make death too easy and quick as well as those that make it too agonizing and prolonged." Professional people can be all too susceptible to the elitism and power inherent in their positions; they can easily slip into the role of deciding these questions for others on the basis of their own opinions of what is best for them (we refer to that as paternalism). They know, but may forget, that the answers are not simple and that there are no ideal solutions. The life and death decisions can only be undertaken with a profound sense of humility and reserve. They raise moral, social, technological, philosophical, and legal questions which in many instances have no universally accepted answers. Indeed, our attempts to wrestle with these issues may be imperfect, but that in many ways defines the human condition. These decisions *should* be hard, because life often challenges us with hard choices for which there are no ideal solutions, and in this, our present situation does not differ from the questions put to previous generations.

The central theme, therefore, in decision-making may be the question of autonomy versus paternalism. Paternalism has been defined as, "roughly the interference with the person's liberty of action, justified by reasons referring exclusively to the welfare, good, happiness, needs, interests or values of the person being coerced."[1]

It has been clear for many years in the law that the patient has the right to self-determination. But medical skepticism of the patient's capacity for self-determination is not new either. In fact, if we look back to the time of Hypocrates (called the Father of Medicine, 400 B.C.) for an opinion about how physicians should in fact control the patient's decision-making, he said, "Perform [these duties] calmly and adroitly, concealing most things from the patient while you are attending to him. Give necessary orders with cheerfulness and sincerity, turning his attention away from what is being done to him; sometimes reprove sharply and emphatically, and sometimes comfort with solicitude and attention, revealing nothing of the patient's future or present condition."[2]

Autonomy, as a legal principle, is not something new. As long ago as 1914, Justice Cardozo, writing for the New York Court of Appeals, said, "Every human being of adult years and sound mind has the right to decide what shall be done with his own body."[3] That's autonomy. In order to understand how autonomy is given effect in patient decision-making we have to look first at a basic determination made about the patient—whether or not the patient is competent. This concept of competent/incompetent does not refer to legal incompetency as would be declared by a court in a guardianship proceeding. This sort of competence is a question of fact, and it's really not very complex. To be considered competent patients must meet two criteria: they must have the capacity to understand the information that is provided to them in order to make the decision and the ramification of that decision; and they must be able in some way to communicate their response to that information. That doesn't mean that they have to be able to write or sign their names on a special form. It doesn't mean that they even have to be able to speak, for after all, communication can be accomplished in many ways—a nod of the head or a wave of the hand may speak just as clearly as written or spoken words.

Once the patient is determined to be competent—and the law presumes that all patients are competent, unless there are significant signs that the presumption is incorrect—then the competent patient has the right to decide for herself or himself whether or not to have treatment. In order to make that decision, the patient must be provided certain information—thus we arrive at the concept of informed consent.

INFORMED CONSENT—THE COMPETENT PATIENT

The basic procedure whereby the patient's right to choose is assured is through the informed consent process. Originally, the informed consent process had its legal underpinnings through the common (i.e., judge-made) law. Basically, if a patient was touched without permission it would be battery. Touching can be anything from a minor procedure such as a bath through a surgical procedure or an invasive diagnostic procedure. Any unpermitted touching would be a battery and would therefore be unlawful. Thus arose the concept of *informed consent.* Basically, the information is required to be provided by the person who is going to perform the procedure on a patient. Usually that is the physician. He cannot delegate this legal duty to any other members of the health care team. The patient has the right to discuss the information, choices, and so on with the physician *himself.*

While the strict requirements concerning the disclosures vary from state to state, generally there are seven categories that should be revealed to the patient to make an informed consent legal. These categories are:

1. Diagnosis
2. Prognosis
3. Description of the proposed treatment(s)
4. Risks, hazards, and benefits of the proposed treatment
5. Alternative treatments
6. Risks, hazards, and benefits of the alternative treatments
7. Risk of doing nothing

We can see that this informed consent procedure is meant to be a partnership between physician and patient. The physician provides the information and the patient makes the choice. Outside the courtroom, surveys of patients and doctors indicated little consensus on what constitutes informed consent. Most of the physicians questioned about informed consent never talked about the hazards and risks of the procedures at all. And patients with whom informed consent was discussed said such things as "It means letting the doctor do whatever was necessary, best or what he saw fit to do" or "giving a person permission to kill you."[4] How ironic that health professionals have sometimes resisted informed consent so strongly, and yet should know that the informed patient who has been fully apprised and has actually exercised his own decision-making in the treatment, often has better physical results than those patients for whom the decisions were made by the health care professionals.

INFORMED CONSENT—THE INCOMPETENT PATIENT

If the patient does not meet the two-pronged test for competence, the information must still be disclosed. If a legal guardian has been appointed, that person alone has the right to make the decisions. However, if no guardian has been appointed, traditionally the medical profession has relied upon the close family members to be surrogate decision-makers. In some states legislation has provided for the family members to consent, even though no legal guardian has been appointed. In the absence of such legislation, technically, the family does not have the legal right to make any decisions regarding treatment on behalf of the patient. However, if there is consensus among the family members, no prior indication that the patient would have made a different decision, and the doctors also agree, no court action will be necessary. In the absence of such consensus, however, the agency and/or the physician may insist upon a court order to treat or to abstain from treating in order to be protected from liability later.

REFUSING OR WITHDRAWING TREATMENT

Overall, with competent patients, the legal right to refuse is as strong as the right to consent. The courts have continually enforced these rights when asked. From dialysis, to respirators, to blood transfusions, to nasogastric tubes, the courts have permitted competent persons to refuse or to discontinue treatment. The right is there, it is grounded in constitutional and common law concepts or privacy, but it is not absolute. There are certain factors that a court may consider to override the patient's right to decide in certain circumstances. These factors are rights of third parties (usually minor children), the preservation of life or prohibition against suicide, and the ethics of the health care professionals involved. These factors must be weighed against the invasive nature of the treatment proposed and the likelihood of success of the proposed treatment. Overwhelmingly, however, the courts have not found these factors more persuasive than the patients' rights to decide.

The incompetent patient shares the legal right of the competent patient to make his/her own treatment decisions. However, the incompetent patient poses certain problems that the competent patient does not pose. The basic problem is, who is going to speak for the incompetent patient? The competent patient can speak for him/herself, but the incompetent patient needs a surrogate to do that. Surrogacy is a significant aspect of many legal decisions, because ordinarily the courts are not the surrogates. With rare exceptions, the courts are not deciding what should be done in a particular case. The courts are merely deciding whether the patient has a right to decide (usually to refuse or withdraw) treatment. The court is not making the decision. The courts did not say "unplug Karen Quinlan; turn off the respirator." Rather, the court said that patients have a right to have treatment discontinued as part of their right of privacy. Furthermore, the courts have usually declared that the surrogate decision-maker(s) must make the decision based upon what they thought the patient would do if she were able to make the decision for herself today. In substituted decision-making the surrogates stand in the place of the patient in making the decision.

Some Examples

Let me introduce three critically ill patients who were central figures in three important legal cases to illustrate how the right to decide is effectuated in health care. The first one was Claire Conroy, an eighty-four-year-old nursing home patient with severe organic brain syndrome and a variety of other very serious diseases: chronic foot, leg, and hip ulcers; urinary tract infections; arteriosclerotic heart disease; hypertension; diabetes mellitus. Except for minor movement, she was unable to move or to see. She lay in bed in a fetal position. Sometimes she followed people with her eyes, but often simply stared blankly ahead. Her general physical appearance was very withered. Ms. Conroy was totally dependent on an nasogastric tube (a tube that goes through the nose into the stomach to enable a patient to eat when the patient cannot or will not take food orally) for nutrition and hydration. Her only living relative sought to have the feeding tube removed, understanding that the removal would result in her death. Both the doctor and nurse in charge disagreed with the decision. Her nephew went to court seeking a decision that it was permissible and legal to remove the feeding tube. The case went through three levels of courts until the New Jersey Supreme Court, in a forty-page decision, reversed an appellate court's decision that it would be euthanasia to remove the tube. The New Jersey Supreme Court ruled that in certain circumstances it would be permissible to withdraw or withold life-sustaining treatment from an incompetent patient. Such life-sustaining treatment may, in appropriate circumstances, include artificial feeding.[5]

The second patient was William Bartling, a seventy-year-old California man with several serious and life-threatening illnesses. He was surviving on a respirator in an intensive care unit (a special hospital unit for patients needing special nursing or medical care or monitoring) because of a collapsed lung, the result of a lung biopsy. Both the patient and his wife requested that he be removed from the ventilator. The hospital and the doctors refused, and the family went to court for an order that the ventilator should be disconnected. This case went to the California Supreme Court which ruled that the ventilator could legally be disconnected.[6]

The third patient was named Sandra Foody, a forty-two-year-old patient with advanced multiple sclerosis. She suffered a respiratory arrest and was placed on a respirator. The family sought her removal from the respirator which would have had the likely effect of causing her immediate death. The Connecticut court ruled that the respirator could be legally turned off.[7]

The legal issues in these cases seem to be similar, centering on the patient's right to refuse treatment. But a family member who has been involved in a similar circumstance recognizes how unique these patients are. Each situation was extremely personal and thereby became profoundly singular in the legal sense as well. Clearly, from the decisions in these cases and others like them and in other states the patient's right to refuse treatment is protected by the courts just as much as their right to informed consent. Ms. Conroy, Mr. Bartling, and Ms. Foody all were patients that wanted to exercise the right to refuse treatment. For each it was certain that the refusal would result in death. Without the right to refuse, the right to consent in meaningless.

The incompetent patient (the patient who does not meet the tests of understanding and communication delineated above), however, is very often comatose, totally unable to exercise his own rights. Thus the courts have examined and ruled upon who will exercise that patient's right to decide, and on what basis. In various cases the courts have authorized either substituted decision-making or objective best interests tests. For incompetent patients who have made some prior expression of intent to accept or reject treatment, self-determination is effectuated by the use of a surrogate decision-maker who chooses "what the particular patient would have done if able to choose for himself."[8]

SURROGATE DECISION-MAKING

How do the decision-makers know what the patient would decide? The courts have relied upon three methods. One is a prior written expression by the patient. This is often referred to as a "living will" and may be a formal document or an informal one. At the time of this writing thirty-six states have adopted statutes, codifying a person's right to create such a document (see living will example at end of this chapter). However, a prior written expression may be relied upon even in states that have not adopted such a statute. The majority of patients at the present time do not have such documents, however.

For patients who have not executed a living will document or any kind of written instrument, the courts have been willing to consider testimony from family and friends about any verbal expression the patient made while still competent and able to do so. So conversations with family, friends, or caregivers can be introduced if the patient expressed orally that he would or would not want treatment in certain circumstances. There is nothing that makes an oral expression any less legal than a written document, but the question of credibility may be raised, particularly if there is conflicting testimony about what the person said or meant by his/her statements.

Often the patient made no clear verbal statements either. Clearly, in terms of decision-making, the time to talk with our families is before the crisis. Many times we are able to anticipate that these questions will arise. The questions of "no code orders" (a doctor's order not to initiate resuscitation measures if the heart should fail—these measures include CPR, electric shock to start the heart, and/or cardiac drugs), respirators, artificial feeding, and perhaps surgery, are often foreseeable. To give the patient the greatest autonomy, the greatest right of self-determination, the discussions must be had early, the questions must be raised and talked about. These conversations are, of course, not easy ones to have. It means discussing terminal illnesses and death. It means acknowledging that the day may come when those life and death decisions will have to be made by someone else.

Other legal devices, created while a person is still able to do so for himself, may be appropriate to allow others to make health care decisions when a patient is not able to do so. These devices are all products of state laws which vary, thus any of these possibilities require significant professional advice. Two possibilities are guardianships and powers of attorney. *Guardianship* is a legal proceeding in which a court declares that a person is incapable of managing his financial or personal affairs or both and appoints a guardian to manage those things for him. A voluntary guardianship is created when an individual appoints her own guardian, either for the present or for a future time when she may be incapacitated and unable to make her own decisions. *Power of attorney* is a written document that gives someone else the power to act on your behalf. A durable power of attorney specifically remains in effect beyond the time when the person giving the power becomes incompetent.

However, if there is neither a written nor an oral expression, the decisions still have to be made. In that case courts have often ruled that decisions will have to be based on objective tests. For incompetent patients who have not left a clear directive concerning treatment, the New Jersey Supreme Court rejected the substituted judgment standard, ruling that, "in the absence of adequate proof of the patient's wishes, it is naive to pretend that the right to self-determination serves as the basis for substituted decision making."[9] Rather, the court adopted two best interests tests and delineated the circumstances under which an incompetent patient might have his/her life supports removed. Both tests involved weighing the benefits of the treatment against the burdens of the patient's life. In Ms. Conroy's case, the court ruled that there was inadequate evidence to satisfy any of the tests for decision-making; nevertheless, the court ruled that feeding tubes and other artificial feeding devices were potentially withdrawable and did not differ significantly from other medical treatment.

Sandra Foody, the forty-two-year-old with multiple sclerosis, was also on a ventilator. Likewise, she had never discussed whether she would want to be kept alive by artificial life supports. However the Connecticut court looked at how she had lived during her illness over a period of twenty years. The court saw that her attempt to live life to its fullest did not encompass a life on a respirator with no possibility of recovery. Her vigor for life was the basis for the substituted decision to terminate treatment.

It is in some way appropriate to realize that these cases have been difficult for the judges involved to decide. The law is often viewed by lay persons as cold and mechanical. Yet these cases demonstrate the judges' profound struggles in making these decisions.

"When we deal with questions such as the ones presented in this case, a certain basic humility and sense of one's own limitations are appropriate. . . . We know that mankind's understanding of the ultimate meaning of life, suffering and death is (and probably always will be) flawed and limited."[10] This judge knew that these are not simple decisions. Society cannot escape the choice process, however, any more than can the families confronted with the daily decisions.

LIVING WILL DECLARATION OF
INSTRUCTIONS FOR CARE IN THE EVENT OF
TERMINAL ILLNESS

I, _____, presently domiciled and residing at _____, _____, Indiana, being at least eighteen (18) years old and of sound mind, hearby willfully and voluntarily make known my desire that my dying shall not be artificially prolonged under the circumstances set forth below, and I declare:

I believe that every human life should be given respect in dying, as well as in living. Therefore, I am free to refuse medications, artificial or mechanical means and "heroic measures" to prolong my dying, and I affirm my human right which allows me to die my own death within the limits of social, legal, and spiritual factors. I do not fear death itself as much as the indignities of deterioration, dependence, and hopeless pain, as well as the effect such indignities would have upon my loved ones.

I believe I have the right to die with dignity—respected, cared for, and loved. I consider as unjust the continuation of medications, artificial and mechanical life support systems or procedures and "heroic measures" when there is no reasonable expectation for my recovery from an incurable injury, disease, or illness. I recognize that this document may appear to place a heavy responsibility upon others, but I am signing it with the intention of relieving others of such responsibility and of placing it upon myself, where it rightfully belongs, in accordance with my strong convictions.

Pursuant to Indiana Code 16-8-11-12(a), 12(b) and 18(e), and recognizing that Indiana Code 16-8-11-1 et seq. (Living Wills and Life-Prolonging Procedures Act) does not specifically provide for all of the following provisions, I direct that, insofar as my condition allows me to comprehend, I be fully informed as my death approaches. I also direct that, insofar as my condition allows me to comprehend, I be consulted in all decisions affecting my medical treatment and the procedures which may be used to prolong my life.

In the absence of my ability to be consulted and give directions regarding the use of life-prolonging procedures, it is my intention that this declaration be honored by my family, my physician, my lawyer, my minister, any medical facility in whose care I may happen to be, and any individual who may be responsible for my health, welfare, or affairs, as the final expression of my legal right to refuse medical or surgical treatment and accept the consequences of the refusal.

If at any time I have an incurable injury, disease, or illness certified in writing to be a terminal condition by my attending physician, and my attending physician has determined that my death will occur within a short period of time, and the use of life-prolonging procedures would serve only to artificially prolong the dying process, I direct that such procedures be withheld or withdrawn, and that I be permitted to die naturally with only the provision of appropriate nutrition and hydration and the administration of medication and the performance of any medical procedure necessary to provide me with comfort care or to alleviate pain.

The provisions of this document shall be deemed severable, and the invalidity or unenforceability of any one or more of its provisions shall not affect the validity or enforceability of any other provision. Whenever necessary and where the context admits in this document, the singular term and the related pronoun shall include the plural, and the masculine shall include the feminine and neuter, and vice versa. This document may be executed in any number of counterparts, and each counterpart shall be deemed to be an original instrument. The provisions of this document shall bind and inure to the benefit of myself and my heirs, devisees, successors, assigns, and personal representatives. This document shall not be affected by my incompetence.

I understand the full import of this declaration and request that all legal means be taken to support my choice.

Signed:_____

Date:_____

The declarant has been personally known to me, and I believe her to be of sound mind. I did not sign the declarant's signature above for or at the direction of the declarant. I am not a parent, spouse, or child of the declarant. I am not entitled to any part of the declarant's estate under any circumstances, and I am not directly financially responsible for the declarant's medical care. I am competent and at least eighteen (18) years old.

Witness:_____Date:_____

_____

_____

Witness:_____Date:_____

_____

_____

Witness:_____Date:_____

_____

_____

This Instrument Prepared by: Donald J. Evans, Evans & Evans, Seven Napoleon Street, Valparaiso, Indiana 46383.

REFERENCES

1. J. Childress, "Paternalism and Health Care," *Medical Responsibility,* 1980.
2. Attributed to Hypocrates.
3. Schloendorff *v.* Society Hospital, 105 N.E. 2d 92 (N.Y. 1914).
4. Lucy Kelly, "The Patient's Right to Know—A Reprise," Nursing Outlook 31 (1983):6.
5. *In Re Conroy,* 486 A. 2d. 1209 (N.J. 1985).
6. Bartling *v.* Superior Ct., 163 Cal. App. 3d 186 (1984).
7. Foody *v.* Manchester Mem. Hospital, 482 A. 2d. 713 (Conn. 1984).
8. *Conroy,* p. 1229.
9. Ibid., p. 1231.
10. Ibid.

SUGGESTED READINGS

Annas, G. *The Rights of Hospital Patients.* New York: Avon, 1975.
Annas, G., L. Glantz, and B. Katz. *The Rights of Doctors, Nurses and Allied Health Professionals.* New York: Avon, 1981.
Ashley, J. *Hospitals, Paternalism and the Role of the Nurse.* New York: Teacher's College Press, 1976.
Cantor, Norman L. *Legal Frontiers of Death and Dying.* Bloomington: Indiana University Press, 1987.
Hemelt, M. and M. Mackert. *Dynamics of Law in Nursing and Health Care.* Reston, VA: Reston, 1978.
Lynn, Joanne. *By No Extraordinary Means: The Choice to Forgo Life-Sustaining Food and Water.* Bloomington: Indiana University Press, 1986.
Mitchell, Mary Harter. *Legal Reference for Older Hoosiers.* 2d ed. Indianapolis: Indiana Bar Foundation, 1983.
Springer, D., and T. H. Brubaker. *Family Caregivers and Dependent Elderly.* Beverly Hills: Sage, 1984.

DEMENTIA

"Is this dementia, depression, or confusion related to medication, grief, or loneliness?" The answer to this question can sometimes be found only through long and careful evaluation—a time full of uncertainties and fear for everyone concerned. This evaluation is most important because, happily, some conditions are reversible. Unfortunately in other instances they are not, and families pull together their resources to help a parent as best they can.

Three personal narratives are presented here by Kitsy, Emily, and Wendy expressing how each individual family discovered and dealt with a parent's dementia. Lisa, who helped us in a conference for caregivers, presenting her "staged interventions for coping with Alzheimer's Disease," addresses issues arising out of these stories. She responds directly to each of these and to Sarah, Karen, and Mary Anne, explaining dementia, discussing common problems and family reactions, and offering thoughtful, valuable suggestions for managing.

Full Circle
Kitsy Beck

I lived with my in-laws during the last two years of World War II and while my
husband was finishing his last two years of college. Those years were ones of
learning to cook, clean a house, iron, and take care of my young son . . . all at
the knee of a rather strict, work-oriented, dominating mother-in-law, who smiled
a lot but showed little real affection. We developed during the next thirty years a
pleasant, distant, and somewhat wary relationship—wary on her part because I
learned to be very assertive and vocally expressive about my emotions, wary on
my part because she was always a real or imagined threat to my close and
confidential relationship with my husband and our five children. I spent thirty-
five years with the feeling that she was in constant disapproval of *something*
about me. So, when we moved back to the midwestern state of our youth and
upbringing ten years ago, close enough to my in-laws to visit more than on
holidays, both Mom and I sort of backed off from each other as if we had to make
room for a new relationship to develop.

Three years after our return to Indiana, my father-in-law, Pop, had an operation to remove a blood clot from his brain and never fully regained his gentle
personality. Now that I am familiar with the symptoms of Alzheimer's Disease, I
realize that may be what he developed. For the next four years, my mother-in-
law took full care of him with a one day per week assist from a niece and visits on
weekends from either my husband, myself, or both of us. She has an older son
who lives in the Far West and comes to Indiana once a year. He seemed totally
unable to accept his father's illness and now is unable also to accept his mother's
illness. Facing reality is not a strong family trait, and most of the relatives
consider me an extremely (painfully) blunt and practical person who has entirely
too much to say about everything.

During the last two years of Pop's life he became increasingly difficult to care
for. He was incontinent, sometimes hostile, had great difficulty walking, and

hardly talked at all. The things he did say made no sense to the person he was speaking to, and "to spare him embarrassment," Mom talked for him, finished sentences for him, talked about him (in front of him), and nearly drove me wild. I thought that, given half a chance and some therapy, Pop could have regained some functions. We began to realize a year before Pop died that Mom was doing some very peculiar things too, but we thought this was because she had restricted her life to such an extent, literally "sacrificing herself on his altar." She had a hard time getting to the store. She would constantly buy things she already had. She never seemed to cook much, and Pop was getting weaker, but of course, we thought this was because he was actually very ill.

He had a couple of turns in the hospital (pneumonia), and the last winter he was alive we brought them both to our house to spend the winter. I was working, as was my husband. We thought Mom would just continue to take care of Pop, and we would do our jobs, then come home and help by getting dinner and getting Pop to bed.

The three months were a disaster. I was furious most of the time because Mom just seemed to give up and do absolutely nothing. More and more she left Pop's care to us, made no effort to help in the kitchen at all, and seemed to "forget" to do the simplest things. I thought she was being lazy and stubborn. I tried to do a little rehabilitation on Pop—getting him colorful kid's books to look at, making up a box of feelies for him because he loved to pick at and pick up everything and rub it between his fingers. Mom snorted her disdain of these kid's toys and happily removed the box from him the day he tried to eat the play-clay. When spring arrived (finally!) she got homesick, and I was happy to help her pack and return to her own home eighty miles away.

By this time, my husband was taking care of paying all their bills and keeping her checkbook balanced, because she said it was just so much trouble. The truth was that she would bring in the mail and simply forget ever to pay the bills or keep track of checks, and my CPA husband was horrified at this sloppy approach to finances.

We resumed our weekly visits, and about a month after they had returned to their own home Pop broke his hip, went to the hospital for an operation and thence to a convalescent home where he died, two and a half years ago. Mom, my husband, and I were with him when he died. He was almost in a coma, but squeezed my hand three times and did his best to smile at Mom and my husband. Mom and Pop had been married almost sixty years and she had hardly ever been parted from him. She took his death with what appeared to be a minimal amount of grief, and we thought that she would now be able to do the things she had given up for the past four years: go to dinner, go to some shows, visit her relatives, and have some good times.

She went through a period of what we thought was normal confusion caused by depression. She went to visit a sister-in-law and spent most of the time there asking where they were and when were they going home. She wanted to stay in her own home, was quite adamant about not living with either son, and although she would come down to visit us for a few days at a time, she always soon got homesick. She began to forget when someone had been to visit her and whether she had eaten. We could tell she had not cooked much of anything, so we got Meals on Wheels for her.

Before long, we saw that she was leaving most meals, partially eaten, on the kitchen table, the counter, or on the living room TV . . . anywhere. She frequently appeared to wear the same clothes for days on end, and although she never wanted me to do laundry—saying she could still take care of things—I was certain from the grimy look of the pillow and unmade bed that she did not change sheets, do laundry, or, in fact, take care of anything. She left newspapers all over her house, piled her unwashed underwear on the bathroom floor, forgot to water her many plants, and made little effort to read or work crossword puzzles—both of which she had previously enjoyed. She quit driving at all, going out of the house only when we or a neighbor took her. She stopped going to church with a neighbor, saying it was just too much trouble, and she literally never called anyone on the phone, although she was always delighted to hear from any of us when we called. She did not write notes or letters and no longer remembered birthdays or any special days until we reminded her, for instance, that it was Christmas. All of these things we attributed to depression and the fact that she was getting older, but they were all very uncharacteristic of her.

Mom had been an alert and interested woman most of her life, keeping up with many friends and relatives, working for years as the head bookkeeper at a large university, doing many crafts such as needlepoint and crochet, working as a Pink Lady at the hospital after her retirement. And always she had been meticulous about her person and her environment. Now she seemed to me like a skyscraper, once full of life and vigor and activity, whose offices were being vacated one by one. I thought I could see her lights going out . . . slowly but surely, and I told some of our relatives that I thought she had just been so burdened with care for Pop that at some point she had gone insane, very quietly, and the result was this peculiar behavior she now exhibited.

A year ago we discussed the possible solutions to what began to loom as a real crisis. I was and still am adamantly opposed to nursing homes. I didn't think Mom could stay in her own home much longer, but I really was not crazy about the idea of having her as a permanent guest in my home either. We toyed with the idea of getting a live-in companion, but they are hard to find and not always reliable. My brother-in-law and his wife suggested a retirement home in a distant town, removed from all of us and from anything familiar to Mom, and I opposed this.

I didn't have the same emotional attachment to Mom that a daughter might have, so uppermost in my mind was how to care for her in a way that would be easy for us and still bring her some happiness. I have always feared being old and alone myself, so when I called Mom and she would say, "I'm just awful lonesome," I felt guilty that I wasn't there instead of here, angry that I had to think about it at all, fearful that someday the same thing might happen to me, and rationally certain that some move needed to be made, and soon.

She was with us for Thanksgiving and Christmas last year, and we took her home New Year's Eve. Five days later she called me. That in itself was an instant clue that something was drastically different because she hadn't made a phone call for about three years.

She said, "Where are you?" "I'm here at home," I answered. "Well," she said plaintively, "I'm somewhere, and I'm in a house, but I don't know where I am."

I knew the time for discussing alternatives was over. "Stay right where you are," I said to her. "I'll be there in two hours and then you'll be safe. I know where you are." I knew at that moment that I was making a commitment to this woman that would change my life. I am not a selfless, martyr-type. I had spent several years arranging my life so it would be "perfect," and it nearly was; but sometimes it is absolutely necessary to do what is decent and human and right, and this was the time. Since my husband had to work, my son and I went to pack Mom's bags and bring her to live with us.

That was almost nine months ago, and it has been a challenge, an irritation, and an always-interesting experience having Mom here. When she first arrived we had never heard of Alzheimer's Disease. We also had not even dreamed of the extent of her illness or the terrible hardship she must have faced living with a dimming and confused mind, trying to keep it a secret, or just not understanding what was happening to her. I think she probably simply forgot all the frightening things that must have happened when she was alone, never remembering to tell us about them. We have been horrified to discover how little she can do or remember.

At first she talked very little, so we only gradually became aware of what mental capacity she had lost. As she became adjusted to being around Al and me and our son who visits almost every day, she talked more and even began to ask questions. She would ask if certain people were dead who were still living, but she never mentioned Pop.

I realized she remembers very little about him, and now she remembers only that he was "a very good Pop." She does not recall the years of his illness or when he died, and I think that's good. The other day she was very confused and asked me where he was. Gently I told her he had died two and a half years ago and she cried and said, "How can that be? How could Pop die before me? I never thought that would happen." But usually remembering or talking about him brings smiles to her face, not tears.

There are many days when she thinks I am her mother, or just a very nice lady who comes in to help out around the place. She never ceases to be totally astonished when I tell her that her son and I have been married for forty years. Most of the time she thinks my husband is her brother, or that Al and I are brother and sister. I am reasonably certain this is her way of writing off a marriage she never really approved of even though she doesn't realize she's doing it.

Mom will get up from the kitchen table to do something, put water in the dog's dish for instance, and by the time she has walked around the table she forgets why she got up. She forgets the way to her room and her bathroom. She forgets which direction the kitchen is from her bedroom, not once in awhile, but daily. She goes out to lunch with Al and me—we try to take her out to lunch once a week and out to dinner twice a week—and then not only forgets that she's been anywhere, but forgets that she's eaten.

My husband took her back to her home town, eighty miles away, to the opening game of this year's football season because she's been going to the games for forty years (and so has he—they are both really structured people). Since it was very sunny she got sunburned. By the time she got home that night, she had totally forgotten the game and had no earthly idea how she got sunburned. By the next day, she had forgotten that her arms were red because they were sunburned and did not know what was wrong with them at all.

During one hectic week she brought in the mail and hid it in a different place every day. She answered the phone, which has a note on it saying, "MOM—DON'T ANSWER THE PHONE," and took messages which, of course, were never delivered or wandered off to look for one of us, leaving my friends waiting on the other end. She put ice cream in the dishwasher, salad in the freezer, dirty dishes in the refrigerator, and let the dog, who is diabetic and restricted to the house, out.

She told two of my friends who came to the house with messages for me that she had no idea where I was (I was in carft workshop in the basement), but she would of course deliver the message. I found out days later that they had been here. She insisted on calling my husband to "see if he's coming up here tonight." She looked up our home number in the book and was going to call, so I just gave her Al's office number and suggested that she call and find out what time we could expect him home. By now, Al and I are inured to the unexpected, and nothing causes the pain and panic that everything caused during the first few months we were getting adjusted to the situation. It is hardest of all to get used to having little or no privacy after ten years of having lots of it! It was very hard for me to realize that Mom was not playing games and to develop the ability to answer every question forty times. I have accepted the fact that the Mom who taught me a lot and caused me many troubled moments during my early married years is gone, and has been replaced by a loving, dependent, child-person in need of a mother herself. My husband can't yet deal with this fact and therefore he can't deal with Mom in the same way I can. I am firm, make her follow certain "house rules" partly for her own safety and partly for my own convenience, and I have clearly established the fact that I am, at all times, in charge. She doesn't always like this idea and once said to my husband, "Is she just in charge of everything?" He assured her I was, and she said, "Well, if that's true, then okay," and she has not rebelled too much since. After trial and error, we have worked out a pretty good schedule and have made some changes that are better for everyone.

For awhile, because we thought it was good for Mom to be on a stable and fairly structured schedule, we got her up at eight in the morning, after which my husband went off to work, leaving me to supervise Mom's breakfast; give the dog an insulin shot; get Mom dressed and ready for the day and occupied with something; try to get some of my own craft-work done; run upstairs several times during the morning to make sure she was okay; get lunch for everyone by 12:30; and do it all over again in the afternoon. I was going crazy! Mom likes to sleep a lot, and trying to keep her out of bed was a thankless task. Recently we have worked out a new schedule. Al no longer comes home for lunch, and Mom sleeps till eleven, which gives me almost the entire morning to do my own work. I get her up for a hearty breakfast at 11:30. She needs to have someone with her to make sure she doesn't wander off from the table and forget to eat, so she and I eat together—brunch for her, lunch for me. She's happy to sit in the sunroom or the porch room and watch children playing, talk to the dogs, check the traffic, look at the clouds. Her chores for the morning are to get herself dressed, comb her hair, make her bed, and put her dishes in the dishwasher. This takes an hour since she moves a lot like Tim Conway when he's playing the little old man.

I check on her periodically during the afternoon, and at three when I feed the dog I visit with Mom while she has milk and cookies, ice cream and coffee, or fruit and cheese.

At five I fix her a drink of Scotch which she loves, and we visit while I'm getting dinner. Evenings she usually watches TV in another room while Al and I talk or get a sitter and go out to dinner. I don't spend large amounts of time with her, and she doesn't demand a lot of physical care, just pretty alert watching. I can hear her walking around upstairs when I'm in my workroom, and I know if she's off her beaten path.

We have removed all phones from her reach, put a dead bolt lock on the front porch door so she can't get out or bring in the mail, and I have labeled all equipment in the kitchen so she can now tell the freezer from the dishwasher. She has recently started forgetting to flush the john, so I guess that will be the next note to go up.

We take her to get her hair done once a week, and there are lot of people in and out of our house, so she is surrounded by activity and life without having to get too hassled by it. We remind her daily why she is here, where "here" is, who we are, what the date is, who she is, how old she is, and who her children are. She doesn't remember, but she always enjoys hearing all the "news."

She doesn't want a companion. She said, "Oh, no. We might get someone in here that you didn't even like and besides, I'd rather be with you. You're more fun." I think that's nice, although I wouldn't always rather be with her! I am determined for Al and me, that our lives and our marriage will stay intact during this time. We do what is easiest for us, even though it might offend some other relatives. For instance, we refuse to have all the aunts and cousins in for the extended visits they would like to make because we feel we are under enough strain without having a lot of company. If anyone wants to visit for an hour or so, fine—but no longer. No meals, no overnights, except of course, for our children and our grandchildren. Mom no longer remembers who most people are, and it's confusing for her to have a lot of people around spending the night. She always thinks she has to find beds for all of them and think about meals, and that worries her.

We have come full circle, Mom and I, and found love for each other in the process. If there is any good in this futile disease, for us that is it. She loves me dearly now, of that I have no doubt, and I have become the mother-teacher— even though my pupil never really learns anything. I have a lot more patience than I had a couple of years ago and have certainly learned to organize and appreciate my time. I don't feel guilty about her anymore, which is a relief, and when the time comes that I can no longer take care of her in our home, then I will release her without guilt, knowing that I really did the very best I could.

A support group for daughters of aging parents, in a distant town, was a wonderful treasure to find and has motivated me to try to start a support group in my own home town. In listening to the other women who are facing this same situation, I realize that my ideas are pretty good and my situation is fairly tolerable, compared to others. The Mental Health Clinic I took Mom to shortly after she came here was no help at all. They were supposed to do an evaluation, which consisted only of a few questions about her name, age, and so forth. Their advice to me was: "Take her to Senior Citizens and spend a lot of time with her. She is obviously dependent on you and you both have a fine relationship." I was looking for a name for what was wrong with her and some ideas on how to cope with or rehabilitate her, not for pastimes or ways to spend *more* time with her. At that time, I was spending all day, every day, seven days a week trying to cope with just having her in my house.

We have recently taken the final and irrevocable step of selling her house and bringing to our house those of her things that we could accommodate. She accepted this with calmness and seems happy to have some of her furniture here. She knows that her mind just doesn't function properly, and we all laugh about it together. I figure if she doesn't cry about this tragedy, why should I? So we just joke about it and tell her if she doesn't flush the john, I'll cut off her Scotch. But she says, "Oh, I know you. You'd never do that to me." If she feels safe and trusting with me finally, after forty years, we must be doing something right.

RECOMMENDED READING

Powell, Lenore S. and Katie Courtice. *Alzheimer's Disease: A Guide for Families*. Reading, MA: Addison-Wesley, 1983.

A Letter to a Friend

Emily

Dear Martha,

Your letter arrived today, asking my advice about taking your elderly mother to live in your home. I suppose the four years that I spent caring for my (now) ninety-two-year-old mother here in my home would qualify me as knowledgeable about the subject, so I will try to pass along some of the things I learned, mostly the hard way—by trial and error.

How ironic is the timing of your letter! After struggling those four years to cope with the same situation you now describe, I finally placed my mother in a nursing home just two months ago when she became unable to walk unassisted.

To make such decisions as you now face will require more raw courage, faith, and strength than you can imagine. Whatever you decide will be a compromise at best for both you and your mother. It is usually difficult for more than one family to live under one roof. If your mother's physical and mental health are both good, then the adjustment to any new living arrangement will be easier for you both. However, you should be aware that as time passes her condition will probably change (for the worse).

You should weigh the circumstances pro and con as carefully as you can before you make your decision. Consider some alternatives—nursing home, homemaker services, help from neighbors, live-in housekeeper. What are your mother's wishes? Are they practical given the circumstances? (State of health, finances, distance of her residence from yours, etc.) Is she capable of making and/or participating in a practical solution?

After working your way through the preceding questions, approach your own family living at home—husband and children—with the same type of questions before you make any decision involving them, especially if that decision involves inviting your mother to move into your home. By all means consult your mother in the decision-making process, if at all possible. Once you have made the decision, go with it! And good luck!

In my own situation, having my mother come into our home seemed the best solution given all the circumstances at the time. Our children were all grown and on their own, so we had plenty of room. My husband agreed with me that having Mother move in with us seemed best for all concerned. Mother's physical health was excellent, but her mental faculties had diminished so that she could not function on her own. Of course, the very fact that she had lived alone, by choice, for the ten years following my father's death, and was able to do so until she was eighty-eight years old is nothing short of remarkable!

I suppose that the loneliness and inactivity during those years that she lived alone played a part in her mental deterioration. As you know, my mother was never outgoing or socially active. I worried about her frequently, but since I lived 120 miles away I was not able to provide constant help and care. However, as an only child I felt an increased sense of responsibility for my mother's welfare as she faced life as a widow. I visited her more frequently, alone, for longer periods of time. I ran errands, did heavy cleaning, and tried to give her emotional support. Several neighbors (including your mother!) were a great help when I could not be there, but basically Mother was fairly independent.

Each year before Christmas I would drive down and bring her to our home, where she would remain until spring. At that time we'd reverse the trip. This ritual was repeated for the first ten years of her widowhood. In hindsight (which certainly is a wonderful thing!) I suppose I knew that if Mother lived long enough she could not continue to live alone at such a distance from me.

I cannot remember when I first became aware that her mental faculties were diminishing, or what prompted me to become concerned. The signs were probably there, but I suppose my mind chose to ignore them. As I have said many times, the handwriting was on the wall, but I kept erasing it.

Suddenly (it seemed) I was confronted with a crisis situation sometimes called "What shall we do about Mother?" As I have explained to you, we worked our way to the decision of having her come and live with us. Considering the "belling the cat" syndrome, how do you tell your mother that she must give up her precious home, her possessions, her privacy, her very self, to come and live with you? Well, you just *do* it, somehow, grieving with her over her lost life, but knowing that you are fulfilling your moral obligation to "honor . . . thy mother."

I will elaborate on a few of the experiences we shared over the four years of Mother's residence here, so if you make the same decision that we did, you may be able to perceive what awaits you. Be aware that these are only *my* observations and experiences. While some may be common and others rare, I found myself called upon to deal with them all. Remember there are no written guidelines to follow. Take each day as it comes; try to keep your sense of humor, your patience, your perspective, and above all, *trust your instincts!*

I think the hardest thing for me to adjust to was the changing dependency between my mother and me: she became increasingly dependent and in need of care and comfort, and I became the caregiver. Neither of us felt comfortable about this, but it was a fact of life. Sometimes (a lot of times, in fact) my heart would ache for her as I saw her lose one more shred of her independence. For example, in the beginning she would bathe herself and wash her hair. Later I took over washing her hair when it became too difficult for her. Soon she needed help getting in and out of the tub; then she needed help with the bath itself. Finally, she could no longer dress herself as a result of her mental confusion. Garments had no rightside or topside due to her fuzzy perception of them. Buttons were a puzzle, armholes a maze, and zippers were total defeat. I think the ultimate embarrassment for her occurred the few times that she was incontinent; having to ask for help under these circumstances made her feel like a naughty child. No matter how I tried to make light of the situation, she was profoundly ashamed of herself. At these times my heart bled for her, but there was nothing I could do to ease her pain. Little did I know that within a few months, all this would change. Then on the few occasions when her clothes would become wet or soiled, she would just take them off and drop them wherever she happened to be! Several times I found her in the living room dressed only from the waist up. By this time she was beyond embarrassment, only puzzled as to what had happened to the rest of her clothing.

She became disoriented as to time and place, and after many futile attempts, we stopped trying to orient her. She asked constantly about her mother, who died sixty-six years ago when my mother was twenty-six years old. It seemed to me as if my mother "stuck" at that age—twenty-six. She never mentioned my father or her marriage; she could not believe that I was her daughter (at fifty-two, I would be twice her perceived age); my grown children, ages twenty-five and thirty-two, most certainly could not be her grandchildren—she simply wasn't old enough! The fact that she also saw her two great-grandsons frequently meant nothing to her; they were just two cute little boys who came to visit.

My understanding of her perceived age also helped me solve the mystery of the "old woman" in my living room. I have a six foot mirror over the couch in the living room. When Mother saw her own reflection in this mirror, she thought it was someone watching her. As soon as I figured this out, I covered the mirror with a large sheet. Then she asked where the old woman went!

Once I understood that she believed that she was a young woman, I could grasp many other puzzling aspects of her behavior, including things that she was unable to tell me. A prime example of trusting your instincts! To reinforce her self image as an individual, everyone was encouraged to call her by her given name, not Mother or Grandma.

My husband was very supportive, cooperative, and helpful in dealing with my mother. I could not have managed for four years without his help. However, just remember that no matter how much help you have, the buck stops with you—the primary caregiver.

Mother had relinquished control over almost everything in her life when she came to live with us. She hung on for dear life to two things she could control—overfeeding her dog and refusing to take her medication. The former nearly drove me crazy, and the latter worried me to death. I fed the dog regularly at the same time each day. She always seemed to be hungry, however, and would beg and cry for food whenever Mother ate. And whenever Mother ate the dog ate—scraps from the table, half her dessert set down on a plate on the floor, bites of snacks, and, unbelievably, coffee! The dog got fatter, Mother got thinner, and I developed an aversion to mealtimes! I finally realized that I could not control her behavior, so I tried to ignore it.

The matter of her medication was a different story—one that I couldn't ignore. I became more aware that she wasn't taking her medicine when I found tablets and capsules in the pockets of her clothing on wash day. Getting her to swallow medicine was a full scale battle each and every time. Most of the time she would choke and spit water and medicine out. Since she was taking only vitamins and aspirin for mild arthritis, her doctor agreed with me that it wasn't worth the effort to get the stuff down her, so she won that battle—no more pills! (Of course, one could not do this—stop giving medication—if an illness and/or chronic condition were involved.)

Do you remember how hard it was to get one of your children, as a toddler, to bed? Well, that was a piece of cake compared to the frequent odysseys with my mother most nights. She would say she was sleepy, but she would jump out of bed and practically follow us down the hall after we had tucked her into bed. She said all sorts of things—such as not wanting to sleep alone. She finally said she wanted me to sleep with her! Upon reflection, I recalled that I did sleep with my mother as a child. Now she wanted me to come to bed with her again. Perfectly logical from her point of view, but not from mine. Here was one point that I would not concede, so I held firm. We tried reassurances that someone was close by, or I would sit in the living room in a chair so she could see me from the door of her room, but most of the time nothing worked. She would walk the hall, her handing running along the walls, or go and sit in the darkened living room until she finally wore herself out and went to bed.

When Mother first came to live with us, I could leave her alone for brief periods, long enough to go to the grocery, for example. The last two years that she lived with us, I could not leave her alone at all. I shopped at night when my husband was home. Thank goodness for my part-time job, on weekends only, when my husband could be at home! I dropped out of society completely; my husband and I did not leave the house at the same time for about two years.

You must realize that for six or seven months before Mother entered the nursing home, her mind was completely *gone*. She had no idea who she was, where she was, who we were, or what hour, day, month, or year it was. She was utterly confused about everything due to some form of brain impairment. She could speak, but she could not carry on a conversation. Most of the time she needed help with everything from walking to eating. In the past I could not leave her alone, now I could not let her out of my sight. Can you possibly imagine the strain upon me?

The wear and tear on my nerves from the hassles of daily life began to take their toll. I was short-tempered, jumpy, had difficulty sleeping, cried easily, ate too much, and became clinically depressed. I knew that I could not continue on my downhill path to self-destruction, but I didn't know where to turn for help. I had heard of a local support group, but I thought the group had disbanded. Finally, my dear son-in-law took me aside and expressed the concern of the entire family for my welfare. I promised him I would seek help immediately. The following day I called the Mental Health Center. I was told by a very sympathetic staff member that the group was alive and well, meeting each Wednesday evening.

At the very next meeting, I was there in spite of my subconscious mind, which tried to tell me that I didn't feel well enough to go. I found the group very concerned, helpful, and nonjudgmental. I must have talked for an hour just telling my story. Apparently not too many people struggle with a situation as bad as mine for such a long time. I said that I hoped to acquire "coping skills" from the group when in truth there were no more to be had. I had truly "run out of cope."

After I digested the information that the group provided, including a copy of the excellent book *The 36-Hour Day,* I came to realize that I could not continue to care for my mother at home much longer. Now the decision was not what to do, but when. I placed Mother's name on a waiting list at a nursing home I had chosen. A bed became available in about one month.

The act of transporting Mother to the nursing home was one of the hardest things I've ever had to do. In her mental state she did not realize where she was going. I did not lie to her, but I told her only what she was able to comprehend. People ask me if I feel guilty for "putting her" there, and I am happy to report that the answer is a definite "no." The only emotion I feel is sadness—the sense of loss surely will be no greater when she dies, for I have already lost the mother I once knew. With her memory gone, she bears little resemblance to the woman who gave me life. When I visit her in the nursing home and see her in cloth restraints in a wheelchair, she reminds me of a wounded bird—so small, so helpless, and so utterly pitiful. She doesn't know me, but she begs me to take her to her home each time I go to visit. I do not go very often, as you can imagine. The visits serve little purpose for either of us.

Writing this letter has been more painful for me than I ever imagined. I suppose with time I will gain more perspective. Right now I don't want to recall these unpleasant memories while they are still so fresh and hurt so much. I hope that the telling will prove helpful to you, dear friend, and if it is, then it was worth every agonizing moment.

Love always,
Emily

Life at the Brink

Wendy

A Christmas visit with Mother was the beginning of a dramatic change in my life and that of my family. I was not aware at the time of the difficult role that I would be undertaking in just a few weeks—a role unique in my life. Little did I know of the anguish, the physical and emotional exhaustion that I would have to endure as I watched the slow death of my mother's mind.

The realization that something was wrong with Mother came during her annual Christmas visit with us. During her stay, her behavior began to puzzle me. For instance, on Christmas morning when our son, Mark, assisted with preparing the turkey, Mother became excessively agitated with him, refusing to speak to him for the rest of the day. One evening she had a long conversation with me, *about me,* but was unaware that she was talking to me. I spent that night tossing and turning as I tried to figure out what was happening to Mother.

Mother never took naps, but during this holiday time at our house, she would nap during the day and in the evening doze off in a chair and awake disoriented. Sometimes she would insist that we put on our coats so we could go home; we were in the wrong house. It was difficult for her to understand that we were in my house.

Over the next several nights it became impossible for me to sleep. During these sleepless nights I thought back to her visit the summer before, when there were no signs of unusual behavior. On the last night of her Christmas visit, I smoked, paced, and stared into the darkness, realizing that she should see a doctor. I decided it would be best for her to return to her own physician rather than see one here. Paul, my husband, made the return trip with me. These trips were always a down time for me, but this one was worse. Mother was very passive. When we stopped for lunch she was incapable of ordering and insisted that I order for her, but she didn't eat anything. When we arrived at her apartment in the early evening, I helped her put her clothing away, and we went out for dinner; again, she didn't eat.

After dinner we visited with my sister, Georgia, who lives in the same community. I told her what took place at my home and asked her to make an appointment with Mother's doctor. Then she told me of the strange things Mother had been doing, such as going to Senior Citizens' group wearing one high heel and one low heel shoe. Sometimes Mother would walk to her weekly hair appointment on the wrong day or at 6:00 A.M. and be very upset because the salon was not open. There were times when she would telephone Georgia at 5:00 A.M., which didn't make Georgia happy. I was angered when she related these strange behaviors to me. Angered, because she knew that something unusual was happening with Mother but had failed to tell me, our brother Jason, or Mother's doctor.

The next morning Mother was not up early as usual brewing coffee. She made no attempt to get up, saying she was ill and couldn't eat. It was painful for me to leave that day. Our trip was very quiet as I had a heavy heart and was deep in thought. Once home, I telephoned my sister repeatedly until she finally made a doctor's appointment for Mother.

Mother called three times the morning of the day of her appointment, concerned that Georgia's husband hadn't picked her up. With each phone call she indicated that she was very ill and had put a nightgown in her purse in case the doctor wanted to admit her to the hospital. After her second call I called Georgia inquiring why Mother hadn't been picked up for her appointment. Georgia said Mother was scheduled for an afternoon appointment, so I asked her to call Mother to confirm the time. I then called Mother to tell her where the hands on the clock would be when it was time for her appointment. From that time on, everything went downhill.

Mother was admitted to the hospital directly from the doctor's office. I telephoned her each evening, but by the third or fourth day she was no longer coherent. The following day Georgia called to tell me that she was starting the paperwork to transfer Mother to a nursing home—the doctor had decided she could no longer live alone. I couldn't believe what I was hearing! How could Georgia make this decision without consulting Jason or me? This was our mother, too. I recalled that Mother had told us, "Don't ever put me in a nursing home." I had done a lot of thinking about what had happened during the Christmas visit and was convinced that Mother was lonely and in a deep depression which I felt could be reversed. I called Jason, who lived in another state, to fill him in on the recent events. Since I lived closer to Mother than he, we decided that I would visit the hospital. I called Georgia and asked her to put a hold on the nursing home proceedings until I assessed the situation. Before making the trip, I discussed my feelings with Paul and our son, Mark. They agreed that if I felt Granny didn't need to be admitted to a nursing home she should be brought to live with us. None of us realized the implications of what we were saying.

I spent three days with Mother in the hospital, and was deeply hurt and angered at what I saw. She was totally incoherent and restrained in bed around the clock. The restraint was used for her safety, to keep her from getting out of bed and falling, which she had already done. I couldn't stand to see her struggling to get out of bed, and my urge to remove the restraint was very strong. We spent a lot of time sitting in the sun room, Mother in a wheel chair and out of the restraint. We talked as much as was possible under the circumstances. I frequently told her that the doctor said she could no longer live alone and asked if she wanted to come to live with me or go to a nursing home. The only reply was "no nursing home." She ate her lunch and dinner in the room, and I found myself testing her. She could read the menu on her tray and any magazine I gave her. Several times while she was restrained in bed she struggled to get up to go to the bathroom and by the time the nurse responded to the call light, it was too late. I saw signs of embarrassment on Mother's face for her "accidents." The fact that she could read and was aware of her need to go to the bathroom indicated to me that something temporary was causing her problem. Her roommate told me that Mother was not confused when she was admitted to the hospital.

Before leaving for home, I called Mother's doctor to discuss her diagnosis, but he was still in the process of running tests. How could Mother be in such a confused state in such a short period of time? I couldn't believe that kind of deterioration would strike overnight.

I began the lonely drive home in a snowstorm. It was difficult to concentrate on driving when my mind was full of questions and thoughts of Mother's future. The questions that haunted me most were why—what happened—how could Mother have become so incoherent and confused so quickly? It just didn't add up. Then, of course, if she came to live with us, how would it change our lives? I arrived home in the late afternoon, physically and mentally exhausted.

That evening I talked with Paul and Mark about bringing Mother to live with us. Since I truly believed Mother's condition was acute (temporary) we thought we could restore her to health. Jason and I had talked about this before, and we both believed that if Mother were to go to a nursing home, she would die very quickly there. When I called him that evening he agreed that Mother needed help. Finally, the ultimate decision was made—Mother was to be with our family.

Since the three of us lived in separate states, I set up a conference call with Jason, Georgia, and myself to tell Georgia that Mother would be coming to live with us. Georgia didn't agree or disagree, but did say, "you always get your way." Jason and I made regular long distance calls to Mother. She was still very confused. Jason and I compared notes and made our arrangements. He would accompany me to help pack Mother's things. Since my home was going to be

Mother's home, and she didn't understand what was happening, we felt that everything should be moved so that she would have something to which she could relate. There was room for her two rooms of furniture in my house if I did some shifting of my own furniture.

I called Mother's doctor to inform him of our decision and requested her records be sent to a local doctor. He told me that she would be released in ten days with a diagnosis of Alzheimer's Disease. I knew nothing of the disease and didn't question him. I did know that my mother was not going to spend whatever remaining time she had in a nursing home.

Later in the week, after the conference call, Georgia called to say she wanted Mother's bedroom furniture. I was dumbfounded, but told her flatly that the furniture would be moved here with Mother so she would have something familiar to relate to. Georgia insisted, again, in a more demanding tone this time. I made the same response, adding that Mother wasn't dead yet. Wham! Georgia hung up.

As the time drew closer to Mother's arrival, I began to think more and more about how my life would change. We had only Mark, a college student, living at home, so I was accustomed to setting my own schedule. I did work, but my hours were flexible. If need be, I would stay home with Mother, although I was sure that once she was settled here she would improve. During the last phone conversation with Jason before Mother's move, he asked me if I was sure I wanted to do this. I replied, "Yes."

I borrowed a van from a friend to make the trip because it had a bed and Mother could lie down on the long return trip. I had never driven a van before and would be driving on the highway and through a large city. I didn't think about this until I had to back the van out of the driveway, but when the adrenaline is running high, you do what you need to do. Jason flew from his home to the airport nearest me; I picked him up and we made the last leg of the trip together. About halfway to our destination, I realized that I had forgotten the key to Mother's apartment. It was already afternoon and I decided not to return home for the key. I knew Georgia had one.

We arrived at the hospital early that evening. Jason and I were pushing Mother down the hall in a wheelchair when we saw Georgia and one of her children come around the corner. As soon as they saw us, they did an about-face. When visiting hours were over, we went to Georgia's house to get the key for Mother's apartment. We received a very cold reception when the doorbell was finally answered. I asked for the key, explaining my forgetfulness, and Georgia said she had already turned it in. I accepted her answer and was turning to leave when she asked me to wait as she had some bath towels and gowns of Mother's to give to me. As she put them in my outstretched arms, she initiated a conversation which became a heated exchange of words. Suddenly she slapped me across the face with all her strength. I was so stunned that I didn't react. She was starting to slap me again when one of her children intervened. Georgia's husband suddenly appeared and ordered us out of the house. It didn't take us long to get on the other side of the front door. This episode created a problem, as Jason and I were going to spend the night at Mother's apartment, but now we couldn't get in. We were both very tired from the long trip and the emotional strain of seeing a mother who didn't recognize us, and we were in shock after the episode with Georgia. We drove to a nearby town and stayed the night with friends.

The apartment manager let us into Mother's apartment the next morning. I knew her and told her about the key. She checked the records and found that Georgia had not turned in the key. Because all the packing had to be done in a day and a half, there was no time to give it much thought. Fortunately, Mother kept everything neat and tidy, which made the task much easier. I left some of Mother's belongings for Georgia that I knew had been designated for her. There were interruptions during the packing session as Mother's friends stopped by to ask how she was and to see if we had any items for sale. The kitchen took the longest to pack. I found that dirty dishes and pans had been put away with the clean. That meant examining very carefully and washing what had to be washed so all kitchen items could be stored as packed.

The next morning the moving company came to make an estimate of the cost, and the move was ordered. The hospital called to inform us that Mother had been released; we were ready to leave after calling the telephone company to have the service disconnected. As I locked the door for the last time, I felt a knot in my stomach. I knew I was closing a chapter of Mother's life, and I felt guilty for moving her out of her home without her complete understanding of what was happening to her. As we drove away for the final time, I couldn't look back for fear of falling apart.

A NEW BEGINNING FOR MOTHER

Mother was ready to leave the hospital when we arrived. An hour and a half into the trip Mother told us that we were going the wrong way to get home. I told her that we were going to my house, and nothing more was said. I was happy to reach home since fatigue was beginning to take its toll. Mother showed signs of weariness. Over six hours was a long time for her to be sitting up after spending two weeks in the hospital. Mother had spent a lot of the trip as "copilot" beside Jason and declined all suggestions to lie down and rest. We had a light supper, and I helped her into bed.

Jason had planned to stay with us for two weeks to help me through the transition period, and I was grateful to him for making that decision as these two weeks became a nightmare for me. Mother would allow no one but me to do anything for her. I never moved without her being on my heels. I fell into bed totally exhausted that first night. Jason shared what would become Mother's bedroom, which had twin beds, so that he could help her if necessary. I was awakened the next morning by Mother shouting at Jason. She was still extremely unsteady on her feet and needed assistance at all times while walking. She had awakened, and he was attempting to help her out of bed, but she didn't want him to help her. I jumped out of bed quickly and took over. This became the normal morning routine for the next two weeks.

I spent most of my time with Mother during the next two weeks. She couldn't be left alone for a minute, because she didn't stay in one place for very long, and she needed assistance in walking. Jason took over while I was doing some of the few household tasks that were done, but if Mother wanted to walk I would have to stop what I was doing and assist her. The only time I felt a slight let-up from this constant stress was during our meals when usually I knew she would be in one place for a period of time.

Jason and I took Mother for her first visit with the doctor a few days after our arrival home. As I was getting her ready for that visit, I felt uneasy while bathing her and taking her dentures out for cleaning. I had never seen Mother naked before, and she had never allowed anyone to see her without her dentures. I felt I was violating her privacy. I accompanied her while she was examined thoroughly. I had her medication with me so the doctor would know what had been prescribed rather than trust to my memory. He said that she would no longer need to take one of the previously prescribed medications. At this point I was not very knowledgeable about medications, their side effects, or why they were prescribed.

During this two week period another problem began to surface. Mark couldn't understand why Grandmother wouldn't allow him to help her. This was the only grandmother he had, and even though she was not the typical loving grandmother to him at all times, he still had strong feelings for her. I talked to Mark, trying to explain that this was a temporary situation, hopefully, and if it wasn't, he would have to learn to live with it. Paul was of no help, and I had little time to spend with him. I was beginning to feel tremendous pressure, feeling like arrows were being shot at me from all sides and that I was being tested to the limit.

As the end of the two weeks neared, Jason called to confirm his reservation for the return trip home. I began to feel as if I was being abandoned; although Mother wouldn't allow him to help her, he did a great many things to help me.

Then the miracle happened! When Mother awakened one morning she was once again the Mother I knew. She was more coherent in her speech and smiling once more although still somewhat unsteady on her feet. Jason and I were ecstatic. This confirmed the strong feeling I had when she was hospitalized that "something" was causing her strange behavior—the "something" was the medication the doctor said she didn't need; she had become toxic from the drug very quickly. The toxicity was now gone from her system. What a day of jubilation! It was an early spring day, and the three of us spent the afternoon sitting outside enjoying the warmth of the sun. We talked about what had happened and why Mother was going to be living with my family. Jason delayed his departure for a week so he could spend time with Mother under better circumstances. We spent a happy week reminiscing about old times. Mother's furniture arrived during this week. She was like a child with a new toy after her bedroom was set up, looking through the drawers, examining things as if this were the first time she had seen them. Realizing that Mother would soon be alone in her bedroom, we purchased an intercom system, connecting my bedroom to hers. (Even with the intercom I didn't sleep well, afraid Mother would fall and I would not hear her.) As we drove Jason to the airport, I felt an emptiness and a twinge of fear as I now had full responsibility of Mother.

We made another visit to the doctor, and he made no change in her medications. Mother was now steady on her feet, could go up and down the stairs with no assistance, so we began to venture away from home. In the "outside world" Mother sometimes made loud, unkind remarks; that's when I wished the earth would quickly swallow me up. Occasionally, I would just walk away, pretending that I didn't know her. Eventually I overcame my embarrassment.

I decided to have Mother's funds transferred into an account here. The letter explaining why she wanted this done was written by me and signed by her. When a great deal of time elapsed without hearing from the bank I contacted my attorney to have him check into this. Within a few days he called to tell me that the bank had been very reluctant to tell him, but the account was closed. How could that be? I wrote to the bank, on Mother's behalf, requesting copies of bank statements and the accompanying checks that we couldn't find among Mother's papers. The answer came and the mystery was solved. The account had been a joint account with Mother and Georgia's husband. Three days after Mother entered the hospital he wrote a check to Georgia for an amount that was nearly all of Mother's funds. The day Jason and I brought Mother here, Georgia's husband called the bank requesting a cashier's check for the balance of the money and closed the account. When I told Mother she cried all day. I had never seen Mother cry before. I was feeling her hurt and my anger. How could a daughter do that? I called the attorney to see if anything could be done to get the money. Legally there was no recourse; since my brother-in-law's name was also on the account, he had legal access.

By this time Mother was managing quite well, I thought, so I went back to work on a part-time basis. I stayed home with her through lunch so she was alone for only two hours before Paul came home. She was dressing herself daily, but sometimes she put her slip *over* her dress or put her dress on backwards. Occasionally she even forgot the dress completely and emerged clad in only a slip. She had a great sense of humor, so I would make light of these times. As we returned to her room to dress again, Mother would hit her head and say "this crazy head of mine."

When I started receiving phone calls at home from friends and my office, Mother would stay busy but shortly tell me to hang up. If I didn't she would start a conversation with me simultaneously, and one time she poured a glass of water on me! I thought answering the phone might help her, but I soon discovered that she would tell callers I was busy or not home. Paul, a professional, received important calls at home. The first time *he* heard Mother tell his caller "he isn't home," things changed. She was no longer allowed to answer phone calls!

That summer I thought Mother needed to have some time with people her own age, a day away from the house and respite for me. I approached her with the idea of going to Adult Day Care and told her about the activities. She made excuses why she couldn't go, saying I was just trying to get rid of her. I didn't pursue this any further, but I was concerned because she was spending too much time in her room. Sometimes she did destructive things such as cutting large chunks out of her hair or spreading lipstick all over herself and her room. I discovered she was using a plastic wastebasket in her closet for her toilet at night. She'd forgotten how to use the intercom.

One day as I was getting ready for work, Mother told me she thought she'd like to see "that thing" I had told her about; she was referring to the Adult Day Care program. Paul was home so I asked him to take her that afternoon before she changed her mind. She liked it and started going one day a week. It was a day of respite for me, as the Red Cross van would pick her up in the morning and return her in the late afternoon. She thoroughly enjoyed this day out, and we continued on a once-a-week basis. Occasionally, I would stop in to visit at Day Care; this is where I met Jane, a nurse and the facilitator for a support group for daughters with elderly parents. Because this was a very lonely time for me, I decided to try the group. In the comfortable, informal setting with other daughters, my story literally gushed out. I didn't feel alone any more. I became deeply involved with the group and relied heavily on it in times of crisis.

Paul could not cope with our new lifestyle. He was little help to me, and our relationship was beginning to develop a chasm. I was so busy meeting Mother's demands, that there was no time for Paul. We no longer went out together, and our sexual contact dwindled. I was too physically and emotionally exhausted for either. We reached a point where Paul would leave the room and find something to do elsewhere when Mother and I came to watch television.

One Sunday when Mother was having a bad day, Paul took his razor, a fold-up sleeping cot and left! I assumed that he had decided to live in his office, but he did come back later that night. Another time he told me that he wanted to talk to me after I put Granny to bed. I felt I already knew what was coming and found that I was right. He told me that if things didn't change he was going to leave, and he would never come back. I thought this was a hard bargain. I did a quick assessment of the responsibility I had undertaken, the fact that Mother could not take care of herself, while he could, and told him to go ahead if that was what he wanted. We talked for a long time about many things and perhaps ended up having a better understanding of each other, as he never followed through with his threat.

My problems with Mark were totally different than with Paul, and I still don't know why these problems existed. I often wonder if Mother had Mark confused with someone else. Now that Mark was in his early twenties, Paul and I tried not to have the relationship of "mother," "father," and "child"; his room was his only private domain; he came and went as he pleased. Mother tried daily to get him to clean his room and make his bed. When Mark brought his girlfriend home, which became a rare occasion, Mother was not nice to her. When we did the laundry, Mother counted the number of shirts hanging on the line, complaining about the amount of work he made for me. She insisted that Mark and his girlfriend were married, so *she* should be doing his laundry and *he* should be living with her. We never convinced her this wasn't true. On rare occasions she was nicer to Mark, which confused him further. We talked about her behavior and I tried to help him understand that it wasn't easy for me either, that he would have to learn to ignore it, but instead he eventually developed high blood pressure.

One evening the last straw fell. I did some extra laundry for Mark while Mother ranted and raved about it. I nearly lost control of myself. Later, when Mark was getting food from the refrigerator, she tried to take it away from him, he talked back to her, and she slapped him. I was furious. Since she was so agitated, Mark and I took her to the hospital emergency room. Mother didn't want to go to the hospital and continued a verbal barrage right up to the hospital door. She had quieted down by the time the emergency room doctor saw her, and he suggested that I call her doctor the next day. We made an appointment with her doctor, and he admitted her to the hospital for testing.

I encountered less mental stress while she was hospitalized, but physical fatigue accumulated from two daily visits and my own schedule. Mother and her first roommate became good friends. The nurses told me that they were like a couple of school girls, laughing, taking walks together, and always wanting change for the candy machine. This roommate understood the disease and was very tolerant of Mother. The next roommate was very ill when she first arrived. At this point Mother missed the companionship of the previous roommate; she seemed to be more restless and didn't laugh as much. At the end of two weeks I met with Mother's doctor to discuss the result of the tests. I asked him when he thought she would be released. He replied that he still had some testing to do and implied that he was stretching the hospitalization so I could get rested before Mother's return.

For my own peace of mind, I called Mother every morning after I knew that she had eaten breakfast. One morning during our conversation she cut me off abruptly, saying, "I have to go now," and hung up. I assumed that someone had come for her scheduled test. Arriving at my office, I found an urgent message to return a call to a friend. I returned the call, and my friend said that earlier that morning she had seen Mother walking in the middle of a busy street three blocks from the hospital and had returned her. Mother was wearing her own clothes, which the hospital allowed her to do on some days. I was frantic! I thought of all the things that could have happened to Mother if my friend hadn't recognized her. I left my office immediately and raced the few blocks to the hospital, becoming more angry with each step. Without waiting for the elevator, I flew up four flights of stairs. I checked on Mother first; she was in bed asleep, fully clothed including shoes and hose. I headed for the nurses' station to get some answers as to how Mother had left. No answers were forthcoming. My anger grew. I proceeded to the office of the Safety Division; their explanation was that she wasn't gone very long! We had a stare-down until I realized that I wasn't going to get anywhere, so I left, slamming the door behind me. My next step should have been to the hospital administrator's office with a demand to see him, but I went back to Mother's room and spent the rest of the day with her. When I left I took all her clothing and instructed the nurse in charge that she was to wear only her gowns.

The next morning, presumably calmer, I called the hospital administrator. I was told that he couldn't be disturbed; anger surfaced again. I told whomever I was speaking to that if I didn't get to talk to the administrator, there was going to be a law suit filed against the hospital. I was given the assistant administrator, stated my problem, said I wanted some answers, and he said they would get back to me. The supervisor of nurses called me back. She didn't have any answers either. I gave up; how can you win? I'm still angry over this incident.

Later that week, as I was preparing dinner at home, Mother called: She wanted me there now! I told the family that they would have to finish my job and left for the hospital. Mother was almost in a wild state and nothing I did had any effect toward calming her; she wouldn't even sit down. She left the room with me close behind, wouldn't let me touch her, walked to the end of the hallway and tried to get out through the fire exit door. I suspect that this is the way she got out the first time—she seemed to know exactly where she was going. I literally fought with her to keep her from going through the door as she opened it, then had to half drag her back to her room. I still couldn't calm her *or* leave her alone to go for a nurse. She left the room with me following her and started her exit again! The nurses' station was at the opposite end of the hallway, but this time they heard the commotion because Mother was shouting at me and came to my assistance. Her doctor was making rounds, heard the noise from the room where he was seeing another patient, came out and indicated to me that he would see Mother shortly. We talked about the results of the recent tests, and he told me that Mother would be released the next day. He ordered an injection to calm her. I went home drained but was sleepless. When Mother came home again she sat very passively all weekend; again I assisted her walking.

On Monday and Tuesday she went to Adult Day Care. I made sure that the driver knew that she needed assistance and called the director to tell her that Mother needed extra help. On Tuesday Mother's feet and ankles were swollen, and at bedtime I discovered that she had been incontinent the night before. She had made her bed in the morning without being aware of it.

Because of this new problem, I sat up with her through the night and stayed near her the next day, periodically struggling to get her out of bed and to the bathroom. She was dead weight, couldn't assist me in any way, and was incontinent of both bladder and bowels. The struggle for me was easier than continuously changing bedding. I called the doctor the next day and told him I thought she needed to be hospitalized. There were no beds available, but finally Mother returned to the hospital by ambulance. I hadn't learned my lesson well from previous experience. She was toxic again! I didn't relate this to the first experience because she didn't have swollen legs and feet before. I thought she had had a mild stroke. I fed her except for breakfast and gave her medications. The nurses began to say, "here comes the magic one," when I arrived, because they really didn't know how to cope with her or to assist.

During this time I was frantic and frazzled. One morning I washed gowns for Mother (she was still incontinent), put them in the dryer and was leaving the laundry room to do something else when I heard something in the drying going plunk, plunk, plunk. I stopped to think a minute about the noise and decided I'd better check because the gowns shouldn't make that noise. When I opened the dryer door one of the cats scampered out. I was upset and checked him thoroughly to see if he had been injured, but he was ok. I couldn't believe I was so preoccupied that I hadn't seen him jump in when I opened the door. Only later did it become a humorous event during a trying time.

After hospitalizing Mother yet another time, the doctor was updating me on her medications when he stopped, took a look at me (I think the stress was showing), and said she wasn't going home but must go to a nursing home. I protested to no avail. My heart sank and I felt sick. I couldn't do it! I still protested but he wouldn't hear any more. I called Jason hoping he would say I shouldn't. He didn't. When I protested he said, "Give yourself credit, you've been able to keep Mother out of a nursing center for a year and a half." Paul agreed with the doctor, because life had become too stressful. Mark was undecided about the nursing home. I had never been in a nursing center before and in my shock didn't visit any the next day to make a choice. I didn't want to; my guilt was at an all-time high; how could *I* do it to Mother? I didn't sleep all night, fighting the torment, asking myself a million questions, and finally deciding on a nursing center close to home for two reasons. I had a friend whose father lived there until he died, and the mother and father of one of my support group members lived there currently. Neither of them had made any negative statements about it.

The next day I slowly made my way to the hospital social services office. Tempted to go directly to Mother's room to steal her away, I reluctantly kept the appointment. We talked, and then the social worker made a call to the nursing center to tell them to expect a new admission. The person on the other end of the line wanted to talk to me so I was handed the phone. She didn't identify herself immediately but asked me two questions, "Does she talk a lot?" I answered that one. "What funeral home?" I dropped the phone and began to weep uncontrolla-

bly. The social worker hung up the phone and sat quietly by until I gained control
of myself. I was embarrassed—I never cry, even over things that are very painful
to me. How could anyone be so cruel? I was totally crushed, already feeling
guilt, hating myself for what I was about to do; the pain was nearly unbearable. I
hadn't come to terms with Mother's disease, and the fact that she was going to
die was the farthest thing from my mind. Time was growing short, and it was
time to finish the arrangements. The social worker tried to make conversation; I
didn't want to talk, so my answers were one word. When I saw Mother tears
welled up in my eyes, so I took a deep breath to control myself. It was agonizing
to tell her that she was going to another place because she needed care I wasn't
qualified to give, but when she got better she would come back to live with us.
The ambulance driver got her ready to leave while I stayed very close to her
feeling totally helpless. I walked with them to the elevator and then to my car. I
began crying again and cried all the way to the nursing center. My feelings
toward Mother's new home were not very good after my initial experience on the
phone.

I didn't know where to go when I arrived at the nursing center so I parked in
the first parking lot I saw and went in the first door I saw. How dismal it was.
There was no one around, but I finally found someone and told her that I was
looking for my mother who was just being admitted. She told me how to get
upstairs. I had come into the building through the laundry and not in the front
door. I hurried up the stairs and thought it a little more cheeful, but not much
since I was not thinking clearly. I finally found the lobby and my heart sank
again. I had never seen a more garish area in my life. I was handed some papers
with a request to sign them while three people stood over me. I said I would sign
nothing until I read it and asked where my mother was. I was told she was in her
room, that they were doing a body check, and that I could see her as soon as they
were through. A body check! My God, what had I done? I read the papers (or
thought I did) and signed my name. If you asked me *now* what I agreed to that
day there is no way I could tell you! I was then shown to Mother's room. The
body check was not completed, so I waited. A body check consists of an aide
going over the total body and recording any bruises, identifying marks, and so
on, on a drawing of a body on a sheet of paper. The aide finally left, and I got
Mother up from her bed and into a chair. I sat on the bed and once again
explained to her where she was, without calling it a nursing center, and explained
why she was there. I left her only once while she was eating dinner to go to the
vending machine to get a cup of coffee. I suddenly realized that I couldn't
remember when I last ate, and needed something. I returned to Mother's room
quickly, and a little later a gentleman came in, introduced himself as Jeff, the
activities director, chatted awhile, and asked me to stop in his office sometime to
tell him about Mother and myself. At eight o'clock that night I reluctantly left. I
talked to Paul and Mark about my painful day and told them that I couldn't leave
Mother there. I agonized all night, continually going to a window facing in the

direction of the nursing center and wondering if she was alright. I decided she couldn't stay there, and the next morning Mark and I went to look at another nursing center. Mark thought it would be okay and I was ready to make a transfer. Then I began thinking of Mother's welfare and decided that I couldn't keep shuffling her around like a deck of cards. I left her where she was.

Continuing to feel that I wanted to bring Mother home, her return became our only topic of conversation. Paul said I could if I felt very strongly, but we decided that I should leave her there for a thirty-day period, give her time to adjust, and then if I still felt the same I would bring her home again. I visited her daily, sometimes twice. It was painful because she was still unsteady on her feet, and she was restrained in a chair for her safety. I would take the restraint off and walk with her, then restrain her again when I was ready to leave. On my way home one evening I saw Jeff in his office and stopped to talk to him as he had suggested. We discussed Mother, her past, her interests, some of the events that had taken place leading up to the present, my guilt and anguish. He suggested that I go away for a week's rest, assuring me that he would look after Mother in my absence. I couldn't do that and didn't. At the end of three weeks she was no longer toxic and could walk on her own again. I went to visit one afternoon and she told me that she didn't have time to visit with me as she was very busy helping Jeff in his office. I stayed for awhile anyway watching her, somewhat relieved because she seemed happy, and I laughed for the first time in a long time. She had a nightgown on over her dress. I commented on this, and she told me it was her work apron. With some relief from my anguish and torment I began to accept the situation a little better and established a new routine for myself.

I relied heavily on my support group through each new trauma. No one else in the group was the caregiver for an Alzheimer's family member, but the emotional needs and circumstances surrounding each member had many similarities. The facilitator, a nurse, armed me with information on Alzheimer's Disease which I studied very carefully. Alzheimer's was not as well publicized at that time as it is today. She was able to tell me why the lobby of the nursing center was decorated in what I considered a garish fashion. It was done in vivid colors because as we age our color perception diminishes. I eventually adjusted to the color scheme and didn't get a jolt every time I came through the front door (yes, I did find the front door!). Jeff also became a source of support for me and helped me through other traumas.

I still hadn't taken Mother out of the nursing center or taken her home. I thought I would do a trial run on Sunday by taking her for a ride in the car and returning her without going to my home. Before I left, I received a call from the nursing center. Mother had left the facility, had fallen, and was on her way to the hospital emergency room by ambulance. I flew out of the house, telling Paul as I went that Mother had fallen and was in the emergency room. What I saw when I reached Mother made me ill, and the guilt surged once again. Her face was a mass of blood; she looked like she had gone through the windshield of a car—torn skin, a broken nose, dentures broken in her mouth, and contusions on her hands, arms, and legs. Paul arrived shortly, took one look and left. After she was cleaned up she didn't look so frightening. X-rays were taken, then she was released, and I drove her back to the nursing center. I stayed with her into early morning of the next day when she fell asleep. I returned to Mother again after a sleepless few hours at home. I wanted her in the hospital until she was healed. By this time she was starting to scab, her face and eyes were swollen, and she was a mass of black and blue. Her doctor was out of town, but Mother's psychiatrist was contacted, and he admitted her to the hospital psychiatric unit. The following week was the only time I felt assured of Mother's safety as this was a locked unit with substantial staff. I learned what had happened *this* time that caused Mother to wander away from the nursing home. Mother was toxic again. Because of her having misbehaved at the nursing center, her doctor had ordered another injection of the same drug that caused her toxicity before. Since I was not monitoring her medication I didn't know that he had prescribed the same medication in tablet form to control her agitation.

This was not the first time Mother had left the premises. I was furious. I thought I should talk to the administrator about a fenced-in area so the residents could go outside *and* be safe, but I knew that I was much too angry to have a civil conversation with that individual, so I took my dilemma to the support group. They felt that I was too angry also, and a group of three members volunteered to take my idea to the administrator on my behalf. Because of their advocacy, a fenced-in area was provided.

In the psychiatric ward Mother was hard to control, but they were better trained than I to cope with it. I was also exhausted. I talked with the psychiatrist daily and learned that he was trying to keep her off any drugs, a "drug holiday" to control her if possible. Toward the end of that week he did have to order small doses of another, milder drug, but of the same class, much against his wishes. Mother was then moved to the regular portion of the hospital for two weeks before being released.

Those two weeks were awful; again, I did everything for Mother. She became physically violent and verbally abusive to the nurses, spent sleepless nights, and wouldn't eat. I was familiar with the nurses and aides by this time, and they shared with me some of the wild things Mother would do. One was angry because Mother had hit her with a slipper. I made apologies to them for her because swearing was something she formerly objected to, but it was now part of her daily vocabulary.

I didn't see much improvement in Mother over the next several months as I had before when she was no longer toxic. I saw swelling in her feet and legs again and complained loudly that this was abnormal and finally got an order for water pills (diuretics) which relieved the swelling. I was now taking her home every weekend and on holidays and took her out for lunch once a week, then to the beauty shop. If she seemed particularly fretful when I visited her in the afternoon, I would take her for a long ride.

After Chrismas that year I was dismantling decorations before I brought Mother home for a weekend visit. The nursing center called to tell me that Mother was uncontrollable and asked if I were planning to see her. I told them I was on my way again! Mother was so wild that even I couldn't control her. She was upset because she had a new roommate that she didn't want in her "house." I was told that Mother had awakened around four that morning, awoke her roommate, and tried to get her out of bed and dressed, so she could get out of her house. I couldn't do anything to please Mother for hours. She finally fell asleep and I returned home feeling hopeless. I began to wonder how much more I could take. I thought about putting Mother in the car and destroying us both in an accident. I came to my senses and realized that with a thought like that, *I* was in trouble. The next day I went to the Mental Health Center for help. I didn't have too many sessions, but in one the therapist asked me if I had any fear of getting Alzheimer's. I hadn't even given that a thought until then. I now joke when I'm forgetful; Alzheimer's here I come—or is that really a joke?

During a visit to Mother's psychiatrist I was told that her regular doctor had increased the amount of medication that he, the psychiatrist, had prescribed for Mother earlier. I asked why he didn't change it back, and he replied that he was in a secondary position. I made him primary by calling the other doctor to let him know that he was no longer in charge of ordering psychotropic drugs (the ones that affect Mother's mind) for her. I gradually managed to get the drug decreased until there were no drugs being given.

I have been such a frequent visitor to the hospital emergency room with Mother that I no longer have to tell them why I'm there. I wouldn't even venture a guess at the number of hours we have logged coming at all times of the day and night. I'm always nervous when the telephone rings at home. After a call saying that Mother has fallen, I jump at the first ring of the telephone for a week. It's amazing that she hasn't suffered more breaks than a broken nose and a fractured shoulder. On one of these occasions she didn't respond to anything for over two hours. I thought, "If you're going to do it, Mother, do it now." A most painful time for me was when she had the eleven stitches taken over her eye. She doesn't seem to feel much pain anymore, but when the doctor anesthetized the area she showed signs of a great deal of pain. I would have given anything if it had been me instead of her. She is a wanderer and has left the building twice after dark unnoticed. One call came to tell me she had been found on the highway by a passing motorist and taken to the police station. I arrived at the nursing center just as she was being returned in a patrol car, unharmed. I tried to talk to her about how dangerous it was to leave her home. All she was interested in was telling me about her nice ride. I felt like giving up. Not too long after that she was out on the highway at night, had fallen, and a passing motorist took her to the emergency room. In one two-month period I had Mother in the emergency room five times. I was beside myself and very angry. It was time to start therapy again. The therapist has helped me to face the fact that Mother is going to die, and she is concerned with how I will fill my time when I'm no longer constantly on the run.

I was still denying the hopelessness of the disease the following Christmas. I thought Mother would enjoy baking cookies. I made the dough beforehand so we would have less time in the kitchen (her attention span is very short). I gave her the dough to roll out and the cookie cutters and only supervised. She didn't know how to do any of this anymore and it became an endless task. Since then I have managed to have a somewhat better grip on myself. I no longer have that intense urge to bring her home on the return trip from the emergency room. She's slowing down and showing increased signs of physical deterioration. I too am slowing down, and the amount of stress I can manage well is diminishing. I'm very grateful for the help given to me by members of the support group, but with a lowered energy level now, I am no longer as active as I used to be.

Understanding and Coping with Dementia

Lisa Gwyther

"She seems like a skyscraper whose offices are being vacated one by one." "The handwriting was on the wall, but I kept erasing it." Both Kitsy and Emily's prophetic comments about their mother-in-law and mother respectively graphically illustrate the sad realizations facing daughters as they observe the insidious changes of early dementing illness.

Dementing illness and its most common form, Alzheimer's Disease, are slow, insidious-onset diseases often mistaken for normal aging, grief reactions, or numerous plausible medical illnesses that may cause confusion. Mary Anne, Kitsy, Emily, Wendy, and Sarah's stories illustrate the idiosyncratic effects of early dementing illness on older women, their daughters, in-laws, and multiple generations within a family. While the daughters describe in retrospect the classic behavior, mood, and personality changes of early Alzheimer's patients, each story is unique. These illustrations serve as a continual reminder that the recognition or diagnosis of a dementing illness is *not* simple or obvious, and each suspected patient deserves a thorough professional evaluation.

Each daughter tells her story within a framework and from the point of view of her unique relationship to the affected older person and other family members.

Lisa Pepper Gwyther, MSW, ACSW, is the director of the Alzheimer's Family Support Program and Senior Teaching Fellow at the Duke University Center for Aging. She is Assistant Professor in the Duke Department of Psychiatry's Division of Psychiatric Social Work. She serves on the Medical and Scientific Advisory Board, Health Services Task Force, Respite Care and Family Support Subcommittees of the National Alzheimer's Disease and Related Disorders Association. She is the author of National ADRDA's popularly acclaimed paperback, *Care of Alzheimer's Patients: A Manual for Nursing Home Staff* (1985). Recently, she was appointed to a newly created National Advisory Panel on Alzheimer's which will advise both Congress and HHS on issues of research and policy.

This chapter will attempt to place the natural history of dementing illness and its impact on families in a chronological framework. I will respond to Mary Anne, Kitsy, Emily, Wendy, and Sarah, using early, middle, and later stages of dementing illness as a framework for understanding the common problems and decisions facing families at these times.

EARLY RECOGNITION

An elder's uncharacteristic behavior or changes in memory, mood, or personality are hard for most families to interpret as a consistent change warranting professional attention. Mary Anne describes her mother's lapsed correspondence, procrastination, inertia, fatigue, burned food, and monotony of diet. Yet Mary Anne experiences trauma in her "sudden" recognition of her mother's incomplete checkbooks and the cumulative strain of her increasingly divided energies between two households. Mary Anne feels worn out, pressured, and inadequate in handling her unpredictable yet noticeably altered mother and their changing relationship. Mary Anne is struck by her own need to respond to this problem as she has to other problems in the past—by turning to her mother for help. Yet, now, the problem *is* "mother." She regrets her hasty labeling of her mother as "lazy," and her harping at her mother to try harder. Both of these reactions are common, understandable responses to a previously competent but recently demented parent.

Initially, Kitsy and her family are the confused ones. "Who *is* the patient?" Her mother-in-law's symptoms become evident only as she cares for her terminally ill husband. It's reasonable to assume that the mother-in-law's symptoms are the result of caregiver stress. Kitsy watches her buy groceries she already has, neglect to cook for her ill husband, and her uncharacteristic indifference to his death. When her mother-in-law "gave up" paying bills, her lack of initiative and her stubbornness are written off by other family members as "playing games." Even her acute disorientation after her husband's death is ascribed to grief. However, her "grief" symptoms are similar to many symptoms of early dementia: forgetting to eat, wearing the same clothes, leaving newspapers and dirty clothes around, and withdrawal from family activities like birthdays, letter writing, church, and visiting. Typical of many dementia patients, there are frightening lucid moments—she calls Kitsy to say "I'm somewhere in a house, but I don't know where I am." Kitsy instinctively did what was "decent, human, and right," responding on the spot to her mother-in-law's need for safety, but *in that moment,* as many other daughters attest, all the arranging for her future "perfect life" went out the window. Once Kitsy's mother-in-law moves in, the entire family is shocked to realize how much she can no longer do for herself. She even forgets her way to the bathroom and whether or not she's eaten. Kitsy does what many daughters do at this point. She reads too much into her mother-in-law's disorientation. Kitsy believes her mother-in-law's confusion of

Kitsy's husband (her son) and her brother represents the patient's inability to accept her son's marriage. In all likelihood, his mother's most vivid memory is of a time when her brother was her son's present age.

Emily, as an only child, recognizes her mother's disability as she realizes her visits to her mother's house are becoming longer and more frequent and that she is assuming more responsibility for her mother's errands, household chores, and emotional support. Her mother's symptoms developed insidiously, but the daughter's recognition seemed sudden in its alarming potential. She grieves with her mother over each loss of independence, but the daughter's sense of family solidarity and moral obligation help her do what must be done. Emily's letter wisely alerts her friend to the absence of written guidelines for taking in an increasingly dependent parent. Emily encourages other daughters to take one day at a time, retain a sense of humor and perspective, and to trust middle-aged instincts and accumulated experience in practical problem-solving. Emily's hints actually describe successful coping strategies for the unpredictable changes brought on by early dementia. She recognizes, with appropriate sadness, that this is different than child care—you can't kiss and make it well. Her mother gets worse and needs more help rather than less help. Yet Emily's perspective helps her to acknowledge the positive aspects of her mother's forgetting—her early embarrassment with incontinent episodes changes to indifferent disrobing in public and gradually just to puzzlement.

Wendy's recognition of her mother's disability is complicated by distance and long-standing sibling conflict, not an atypical scenario for many mobile professional families. Her mother's symptoms and stormy course have a profound impact on multiple generations in her family, and yet, as Wendy quickly assumes the role of primary caregiver, she becomes the most vulnerable. Typical of many retrospective family descriptions, Wendy's realization that something is wrong with her mother occurs during her annual Christmas visit. Her sister lives closer to her mother, and she has probably noticed these symptoms for some time, but sibling responses often differ in response to the same situation. It never occurs to her sister to seek medical attention. It's also common for dementia victims to look much worse during stressful family reunions or changes in routine associated with holiday visiting. Dementia patients are likely to fatigue more quickly, often from trying to cover their deficits and live up to previous expectations.

Wendy realizes her mother is "talking to me about me." Her mother dozes off and wakes up disoriented, asking to go home—"this is the wrong house." She can't order or make a decision in a restaurant. She goes out with different shoes on, or leaves for a beauty shop appointment at 6:00 A.M. on the wrong day. Wendy finds dirty dishes in her mother's previously immaculate kitchen. Wendy and her brother go through the usual litany of suspected causes—the effects of a recent hospitalization (which is always traumatic for dementia victims), depression, and drug reactions. Wendy is convinced her mother's behavior is caused by something acute and reversible because her mother can still read and uses the toilet. Actually, reading is preserved much longer than comprehension, and incontinence is usually a much later symptom of dementia.

Old sibling rivalry is aroused by the necessity to protect their mother. Wendy resents being excluded from the nursing home decision, just because she lives away. Sadly, her decision to act is interpreted by her sister as "always getting her way." Just as all the other daughters, there is no way for Wendy to fully understand the impact of her decision to take her mother home, but she aptly explains it with "when the adrenaline is high, you do what you need to." Her mother's move illustrates the symbolic meaning of personal possessions. Wendy's sister may want the mother's furniture because she is losing control of her mother's life. Yet Wendy wisely recognizes that the familiar objects may be critically reassuring in helping her mother cope with relocation.

Sarah, too, is shocked when her mother asks her if she's ever had children. Her mother insists she's never lonely, but this same mother can't bear to have Sarah out of her sight. Her mother's intense fears of abandonment force her to sit with the family through TV shows beyond her comprehension. Ironically, as her mother's shadowing increases, Sarah feels more isolated and alone. Sarah's daughter, Karen, can often get her grandmother to do things she stubbornly refuses to do for her daughter. Dementia patients are often most suspicious and difficult with those closest to them.

Karen's story illustrates the genuine practical and emotional help that can be offered by secondary family caregivers. At first, Karen feels frustrated, guilty, and angry at her grandmother's intrusion. Karen is frightened as her mother becomes more withdrawn, vulnerable, teary, and preoccupied. She recognizes with her mother how scary and stressful it is to become responsible for someone else's body. Their mutual inability to please the grandmother makes them feel inadequate and out of control. Although there is no right time to face these multiple losses and the necessity of increased intergenerational interaction, they survive and learn valuable coping strategies to share with others in their support group.

All these early recognition experiences illustrate the commonalities and unique twists in caring for parents with dementing illnesses. Recognition of an insidious dementia *is* traumatic, and it is generally precipitated by a family crisis. Recognition often forces a decision made under pressure, precluding planning and emotional preparation. The demented parent *is* realistically dependent and care can't be forestalled. While this is normative and stressful, it is possible to make decisions without regret. Once one becomes a primary or secondary caregiver, your life can become shaped by the events of the illness. In dementia care, one is forced to become vigilant and hyper-alert to unpredictable, but almost inevitable crises. The inevitable family adjustments are both concrete and emotional, with the latter much more difficult and time-consuming than the former.

What families in this early recognition phase need most are adequate diagnostic facilities with experienced professional staff. Diagnostic centers must accommodate scared, agitated, suspicious, and unwilling patients and their families in a manner that won't exacerbate the patient's suspiciousness or intensify family conflict. Health professionals must listen and probe the history and symptoms carefully, responding individually to patient, family, and even employer questions. Many families need help telling the patient about the diagnosis, or help with explanations for other relatives, friends, neighbors, or employers. Family fears and sadness over the loss of future interdependence should be addressed. Many families deny and seek cures in health food stores or multiple second opinions. Many families have a need to assign blame, for example, "if only Dad didn't nag her," or "if only she had refused that hysterectomy." Some daughters are shocked to learn their well parent has been covering up the patient's deficits for years in order to "spare the children." Some frightened families come to diagnostic centers frantically coaching the patient on common mental status questions, for instance, "Come on, Mom, we just talked about *President Reagan* on the way over here!"

It's very hard to watch someone you love lose a lifetime of skills, personality style, and eventually even recognition of you. Many families need individual help making sense of the diagnosis and prognosis, for example, "How could she be sick? She never smoked, and she even jogged. In fact, she was the Rock of Gibraltar. Is she just manipulating us? Why is she so indifferent to my pain or the sacrifices I'm making on her behalf? How can I help her avoid embarrassment?"

At the time of diagnosis families should make the doctor aware of their previous and current caregiving responsibilities. Most family members vividly remember both positive and negative experiences caring for other frail relatives, and most are unwilling to repeat bad experiences. The physician should be aware of the caregiver's health status and her other family or work commitments. Some of the daughters in this book mentioned other common commitments like divorced children, children in college, husbands demanding more nurturing, or careers on hold. Most families need help collecting relevant history and understanding why tests are necessary, why questions about the patient's function are so critical, and how medications and other illnesses can affect behavior just as much as a primary dementing illness. It's difficult for most families to take in all this information in a single diagnostic visit. Often the patient is agitated and eager to leave, or the family is emotionally unprepared to confront such devastating news. Families tell horror stories about being told the diagnosis in a busy waiting room, on the phone, or with some clincher like "Take her home and love her—you don't need to bring her back here, we have nothing to offer."

Written materials and referral to local support groups can be invaluable. Several daughters admitted that it was therapeutic just to seek information or to try a support group meeting. Written materials can be digested in manageable doses after everyone calms down. They provide a common family understanding that is an absolute prerequisite to future cohesive family decisions about appropriate care. Many people misread or misinterpret something about dementia, and written materials, plus individualized help interpreting them, can clear up some of these frightening misconceptions. Families must be prepared for the variation and ambiguities in patient function—what the daughters call "the good days/bad days scenarios." Some families need help altering expectations of the patient and help modifying the home to work *for* rather than against the patient's disability. Handling money and driving become immediate early concerns. Families also appreciate professionals who point out the value of durable powers of attorney. When a responsible daughter takes over the bills, there is no unnecessary loss of valuable patient assets. Finally, daughters appreciate health professionals who will stand by them throughout the course of a degenerative illness. It is reassuring just to know that expert, hopeful, and interested professionals recognize your role in caring for your parent.

THE LONG HAUL: FROM MILD TO MODERATE DISABILITY

"I miss the mother I always knew, and I miss being my real self with Mother." Mary Anne's summary of the role transitions and grief reactions to dementing illness illustrates the prolonged nature of necessary adjustments. Mary Anne mourns the loss of a mother who always remembers birthdays, as she simultaneously walks a tightrope between tactful and demeaning responses to her mother's constant repeated questions. What Mary Anne thought was her mother's "temporary need" became increasingly open-ended dependency. This is the very nature of dementing illness.

But Mary Anne gains valuable insight and learns important survival skills. As she watches her mother's physical therapy, she gradually recognizes that it is her mother's *memory loss,* not her loss of physical function, that slows her progress in walking. Mary Anne learns to adapt the environment for her mother, rather than vice versa, and the toilet and shower are modified to enhance safety and ease of assistance. Mary Anne learns that she must do simple tasks one at a time with her mother, slowly enough to avoid "overloading the circuits." Most important, Mary Anne learns how to delegate and prioritize tasks.

Mary Anne's mother is energized only when she feels she is helping someone else. This vestige of her mother's former reciprocal relationships encourages Mary Anne to involve the rest of her family. Mary Anne learns her ten-year-old can take great pride in helping her grandmother. Mary Anne's mother's repeated calls about the date can be handled with a little consumer advocacy. Now their local Weather Line recording offers time, temperature, *and* date. Mary Anne hires a cleaning and laundry helper, lowers her own standard of housekeeping, and saves her energies for chauffeuring, organizing, shopping, and taking her mother out to eat, since it seems to improve her appetite. Mary Anne's children are encouraged to tend grandmother's plants, and to fix things for her, as Mary Anne recognizes how much their task-oriented visits satisfy their grandmother's need for emotional nourishment. Mary Anne's husband flourishes as the objective problem-solver. Mary Anne even reorganizes her own routine for a quiet hour before her family awakes. She exercises, listens to tapes, cooks, and treasures the personal time to reflect. Although Mary Anne, as an over-achiever, is bothered by how much she *isn't* accomplishing, she realizes that much of her guilt comes from comparing herself to her mother. Her mother *never* took time for herself, but Mary Anne wisely recognizes that her needs are different.

Mary Anne's success in handling her mother's increasing dependency becomes her legacy for her children. Her children gain skills and ideas to assist and compensate for an elder's increasing memory loss, for example, different colored boxes with the A.M. pills and P.M. pills enclosed, taking advantage of the elder's best time in the morning for exercise, encouragement of fluids, and showering. From Mary Anne, her children learn to fill in the blanks in their grandmother's elusive thoughts, the importance of tact and patience, and how essential it is to offer needed help to those realistically disabled by loss of adult thinking capacity. They learn they can adapt "treats" to their grandmother's increasing insecurity. (A birthday fireworks show for grandmother is arranged for *indoor* viewing.) Finally, Mary Anne learns to savor successful moments such as a telephone conversation overheard between her daughter and her mother: "Today is Thursday, Gram. . . .Better turn the calendar to Thursday. . . . Does it say Thursday now? . . . Good! . . . You're welcome. Good-bye, Gram."

Emily describes the long haul by saying "the dog got fatter and Mom got thinner." She, like Mary Anne, learns to prioritize. The battles about overfeeding the dog are fruitless, but her mother's nutrition is important. With the doctor's support, she gives up the battle over vitamin pills but doesn't retreat on the issue of sharing a bed with her husband, *not* her mother. She discovers tricks that help her mother relax and feel more secure at bedtime, but resists her mother's demands to have her daughter with her all the time. She learns to modify the environment to be less scary for her mother (e.g., by covering mirrors whose "old lady images" create confusion and fear). Emily, too, is blessed with a supportive family, but she quickly learns that the buck stops with the *primary* caregiver. Emily fights the loss of her identity by holding fast to her part-time job. Eventually, she wisely recognizes that it is time to consider placing her mother when she finds herself "running out of cope."

Sarah and her daughter Karen find answers for the long haul through their support group. A progressive dementia forces family caregivers to become "case managers" in seeking services and solutions. As family caregivers become weaker, more tired, confused, and at a loss, they hopefully come to understand that it is a sign of strength to acknowledge a need for help. Initially, attending the group together provides some protected and shared time off for Sarah and Karen. Gradually, their participation helps them expand and enrich their support network. They become part of a growing constituency of family caregivers teaching each other valuable skills and developing their own insights. They learn practical care tips, such as the value of routines. They make sure Sarah's mother gets to church, the beauty shop, and out to lunch on a scheduled basis. As a family and as a support group, they grieve, reviewing good *and* sad times, but generally succeeding in turning their crises into more manageable situations.

Sarah discovers the value of personal time off, and she arranges it with help from a day care program for her mother. Evenings out with her husband are built in later. Gradually, Sarah is able to take pride in a job well done, and successfully retains her sense of humor to keep their tragedy in perspective.

In the context of the support group, Karen begins to appreciate the variability among disabled elders, who, in spite of disability, still thrive on opportunities to give as well as receive. Even Karen, as a secondary caregiver, comes to appreciate how adjusting medications in a confused elder takes time, trial, error, and a willingness to modify expectations of "living better through chemistry." Gradually, Karen comes to accept her grandmother, not for what she used to be, or for what Karen wishes she would be, but for what she is.

As Kitsy's mother-in-law becomes increasingly bizarre and dependent, Kitsy's image of her changes from one of a disapproving mother-in-law to a loving dependent older woman. She watches her mother-in-law hide the mail, wander aimlessly, store ice cream in the dishwasher and the dirty dishes in the refrigerator. She finds herself becoming increasingly vigilant in trying to head off or predict the next disaster. Much to her surprise, Kitsy learns that care for moderately demented patients is probably more supervision and protection than actual physical care.

Kitsy, like Mary Anne, learns to adapt schedules to suit herself and to accommodate the elder's needs. Her mother-in-law sleeps late, and they eat together at noon. Kitsy gradually realizes that, for her mother-in-law, watching the street scene from the window is a sufficiently enjoyable and stimulating daily activity. This schedule protects some personal time for Kitsy, while still meeting her mother-in-law's needs for attention. Kitsy develops real survival skills to cope with her mother-in-law's increasing agitation in the late afternoon—often referred to as sundowning in Alzheimer's patients. The antidote to sundowning in Kitsy's home is to fix her mother-in-law a scotch while Kitsy makes dinner. They learn, as a family, to deadbolt the door and limit the patient's access to the telephone. Even daily orientation hints for her mother-in-law seem welcome as "news." They learn to limit family entertaining when they realize how agitated her mother-in-law becomes when she tries to fulfill old hostessing obligations.

Much to both Kitsy and her mother-in-law's delight, they find it is possible to discover love for each other as the dependency balance is changed. For the first time, Kitsy is able to gently teach her mother-in-law, and for the first time in forty years, she feels accepted and trusted by her. The support group changes Kitsy's perspective as well. When she compares her situation to others, her mother-in-law doesn't seem so tough!

Wendy's long haul is like an extended roller-coaster because her mother changes acutely with each toxic reaction to a medication. First, Wendy must cope with her mother's stubborn preference for only Wendy to assist with personal care. Although Wendy's brother is supportive, he can't alleviate Wendy's discomfort in seeing her naked, once-powerful mother. Wendy's part-time job helps her recognize the value of respite, and she gradually insists on her mother's regular attendance at day care.

Her mother's dementing illness has profound effects on Wendy's whole family. Wendy's social, and even sexual, life with her husband almost disappears. Her husband threatens to leave before everyone begins talking about what has happened to them as a family. It's especially hard for Wendy to see her mother treat her son and his girlfriend so poorly. Wendy's family's anger about their situation is easily projected to professionals when her mother is frequently hospitalized. It's hard to accept that a familiar trusted institution like a hospital can't guarantee perfect safety for a wandering, confused, and suspicious older woman. Wendy found her skills in dealing with her mother were invaluable to hospital staff—so invaluable that her time and energy are further consumed when staff "let her" take over, rather than learning to substitute for her in her absence.

Wendy realizes she is in trouble when she is preoccupied to the extent of missing her cat's presence in the dryer. Yet, like many other families who easily lose perspective in prolonged crises, a decision about nursing home placement is initiated only when a wise physician observes obvious deterioration in the primary family caregiver. And it is Wendy's brother's gentle reminder of what *has* been accomplished in keeping their mother at home, which comforts Wendy as she faces the inevitable.

What conclusions about the effects of the long haul on patients and families can be drawn from these stories? As with any other situational stress, there are potential losses and gains. Objectively, as dementing illness progresses, safety issues make increasing supervision a certainty. All these families recognize the patient's increasing vulnerability in remaining on her own, but decisions about where and when a patient can be safely left alone vary in every situation. All these families notice alarming increases in behavior, mood, and sleep problems as the disease progresses. The damage to the brain in dementia causes patients to behave in ways they generally wouldn't choose. However, understanding that these changes aren't intentional or willful doesn't make them any easier to accept.

Family caregivers become increasingly fearful as the disease progresses. Each telephone ring may spell disaster or another irritatingly repeated question. Each daughter must face crushed expectations about the anticipated freedom of this time in her life, and each must face increasing helplessness in pleasing her mother, her family, and sadly, even herself. All these daughters express frustration when carefully conceived plans and strategies fall through, or when friends or other family members fail to live up to expectations for support. Daughters are often shocked by the depth of their own anger and their simultaneous grief and fatigue. Yet, these same committed daughters feel continual guilt about what they are *not* doing. Their increasing isolation from old friends and formerly trusted family members seems to increase their symptoms of stress. Some become more vulnerable to their own idiosyncratic health problems. Then, just when they need the most support, they notice increasing family conflict. Differing access to or understanding of information means that other family members will perceive the patient's ability or disability in different terms. These daughters are even attacked by distant relatives for catastrophizing or infantilizing their realistically dependent mothers. Their guilt expands as old promises, cultural, family, or religious rules are thrown in their faces. And often they are forced, for the first time in their lives, to seek outside help.

Asking help of physicians is usually most comfortable, but finding a knowledgeable physician willing to provide continuity of care is often difficult. Chronic illness can be as frustrating and time-consuming for physicians as it is for families, and many physicians don't realize how much can be done to improve a patient's function. Constant monitoring and reassessing medication is inevitable, and it may be more art than science. Treating infections, correcting sensory loss and dentition may not only improve function, but also enhance quality of life for many dementia patients and their families. Finding a primary care doctor with whom a family can work can play a major role in coping with dementia. Often it's the doctor who first recognizes and insists on caregiver respite, and this medical prescription to take care of oneself is very helpful for guilty daughters. Unfortunately, a chronic illness like Alzheimer's doesn't preclude a patient from getting other illnesses requiring emergency treatment or hospitalization. It's important for families to know in advance with which hospital their doctor is affiliated, and how he or she will handle falls, accidental poisonings, heart attacks, strokes, or a recurrent cancer.

Families need specific information and referral from a trusted professional before they go off in search of help. They should know what to expect in the course of dementing illness, and what services might be useful and available. Unfortunately, some daughters, like Kitsy, must still contend with mental health professionals who use cheerleading tactics to encourage family caregivers to persevere. Many mental health providers become blinded by their setting and may not be aware enough to suspect organic illness in a mother brought in by her exasperated daughter for what superficially may appear to be a relationship problem. Many families are further frustrated by mental illness labels such as "pathologic family." This labeling leads to wasted precious time in *un*successful insight-oriented family therapy. Expecting a dementia patient to participate in insight-oriented therapy just frustrates his or her limits of recent memory.

Much helpful informal counseling comes from mutual support groups like DEBUT. Families of Alzheimer's patients have a national organization with an impressive network of 160 chapters and over 1,000 local support groups. The Alzheimer's Disease and Related Disorders Association (ADRDA) is a national voluntary health organization providing, through its chapters, an impressive array of patient and family education materials, media public awareness materials, and opportunities to join legislative advocacy efforts to assist both patients and caregivers. For example, families having difficulty with Social Security claims may use an impressive kit from ADRDA outlining how to apply for disability and how to document progressive cognitive impairment. Some families need specialized information to help children or private sitters understand the patient's bizarre behavior and language changes. All these materials are available through ADRDA chapters and their affiliated support groups. Most important, daughters meet others who can understand, as only one who has cared for a relative with progressive dementia can understand.

All the daughters experienced some betrayal by friends, as they were forced to assume more family responsibilities. Long explanations to casual friends drain a caregiver's energies, which are necessary for more immediate concerns. Caregivers need both friends *and* professionals who understand immediately, and who realize they are not exaggerating the chaotic nature of their lives. Support group members help each other validate what excellent care they are offering. Support groups provide role models—people who have survived care responsibilities with their sanity and integrity intact. These survivors can be powerful antidotes to the helplessness and futility one feels in providing care for someone who continues to get worse. The practical tips and coping skills learned in these groups enhance competence and knowledge, helping caregivers regain a sense of control of their destinies. Knowledge is power, and the invaluable consumer information shared among support group members helps each member make the best choices for her relative's care.

All these daughters recognize their need for time off from the constant supervision and responsibility. Most respite is provided informally, with other family members and friends standing in for the primary caregiver or taking the patient out so the caregiver can have time alone at home. Some church groups offer informal respite to their homebound members. There are also more formal services offering caregiver relief. Some home care agencies have trained aides or nurses available, depending on the level of skill needed. Wendy and Sarah successfully use day programs, which offer the added bonus of stimulation and support for the patient as well as respite for the caregiver. Day programs are not available in all areas, and some program directors are reluctant to take too many confused participants at one time. For some families transportation and/or escort becomes problematic with day centers.

The biggest barrier to caregiver respite is usually the caregiver. It's scary to turn a beloved relative over to strangers, particularly when other disapproving relatives are looking over your shoulder. Most dementia patients lack initiative. They never want to do anything new. But, if they are accompanied to day centers at first and offered lots of reassurance, many will enjoy the scheduled day program activity. Most families learn that dementia patients adjust better to day programs if they think they are there "to help others," rather than to be helped. Dementia patients often don't see themselves as dependent or as sick as they see their more physically frail peers.

Finally, there are institutional or residential respite options in some communities. In "the good old days," doctors would admit frail elders to the hospital when the family caregiver needed a break. Medicare regulations no longer permit these "social admissions." More importantly, geriatricians are learning that hospitals can be dangerous and frightening places for functionally impaired older people. Now, some small group homes also offer temporary admissions for family vacations or emergencies, and some nursing homes or special wings of state, county, or VA hospitals are beginning to experiment with "respite beds" set aside for these temporary admissions.

All these options help families committed to home care continue to care for their relatives and themselves. Successful coping with a long-term illness necessitates a variety of flexible, affordable respite options. No single individual or willing saintly family can offer quality long-term care forever, without occasional time off.

Eventually, however, nursing care needs predominate, and vigilant attention to troublesome or risky behavior becomes less an issue. Some families find this change to nursing care more harrowing than anything else.

TERMINAL CARE: DREADED DECISIONS

Alzheimer's is just one of many ways of dying. It happens to be one that allows a family to say good-bye.—Dorothy Stoneman, ADRDA (Eastern Mass. 1986)

When Emily's mother was no longer able to walk unassisted, Emily is forced to make a decision about placement because she "runs out of cope." Emily describes her mother at this time as "wounded, helpless, and begging strangers to take her home." For Emily, this is the worst part of her mother's illness. Fortunately, the DEBUT group linked her to sources of information. Her reading and talking with others convinced her that the issue was not *what* to do but *when* to do it. Although, with time, Emily developed a healing perspective, nothing ever seemed as painful as the placement decision and the immediate aftermath of transition.

Duke research on Alzheimer's caregivers came to conclusions very similar to Emily's. There is no right time for placement, and placement decisions seem to have little to do with the severity of the patient's illness or symptoms. While an event such as a fall or infection requiring hospitalization may trigger a sudden decision, placement decisions are more often determined by the circumstances of the caregiver and the context of care. Role overload predicts placement, particularly among daughters with high levels of stress and unsatisfactory amounts and quality of family support. Sadly, there is also *no* evidence that institutionalization of a parent leads to an immediate relief of caregiver burden. While Emily experienced relief from the physical demands of care, there was no emotional relief from her responsibility for her mother. The buck stops with the family. Daughters may feel even more overwhelmed because they retain this ultimate responsibility, but they lose control of daily care. Although daughters are more likely than spouses to experience role overload and to place a parent, their well-being often plummets to new lows before they begin to trust the institution and change their perspective.

Unfortunately, recent demographic changes mean more daughters will be facing these decisions between equally unattractive terminal care options. More Americans are not marrying or are not staying married. Americans are having fewer children, deciding to forego child-bearing or putting off child-bearing until later in life. More mid-life daughters are in the work force, and we can assume that many more future Alzheimer's patients will lack the range of family caregivers available to current patients. Institutional options will not go away—nor should they. But daughters will continue to need support and information in facing these decisions. Their families and communities must be educated about caregiving—its contributions, the toll it takes on daughters, and the possibilities for effective local support and services.

Wendy's experience with her mother's placement is almost prototypical. There was no time for a careful review of options and a family conference. Wendy had put off looking at available care facilities despite her mother's frequent hospitalizations. Through all her mother's moves, Emily had become the consistent figure, and to consider placement seemed like betrayal. Wendy's introduction to nursing home care only confirmed her worst fears. She called from the hospital rather than visiting, and the first questions from the nursing home admissions officer were about preferred funeral arrangements! This triggered a flood of grief and embarrassment which understandably precluded rational decision-making. Fortunately, by the time her mother moved, Wendy was able to say, "You need care that I'm not qualified to give. When you are better, you will come home." While this is *not* a fair promise to a competent parent, an Alzheimer's patient is looking for reassurance that she won't be abandoned. She will most likely become aware of her surroundings, and she may forget the promise to bring her home. For now, this is a comfortable compromise for both Wendy and her mother.

For Wendy and many other daughters, the hardest part of placement is the long adjustment period. Her mother wandered and fell, occasioning frantic calls to Wendy's home at night. Again, there was no relief from the constant hyper-alert waiting for catastrophe. The garish lobby didn't reflect her mother's style, and it made Wendy even more uncomfortable. Problems with adjustment to a roommate were embarrassing for Wendy and frightening for her mother. It was painful to watch her mother's "body check" and to see her mother physically restrained. All these situations confirm a daughter's worst fears of retribution for "imprisoning" a parent. Wendy's hopelessness increased as she frantically tried to take her mother out of the facility for long rides or visits. She knew she needed help when she considered running the car off the road.

Gradually, Wendy realized that she was slowing down as her mother slowed. As she slowed down, she began to appreciate the staff's helpful responses to her discomfort. Jeff, the social worker, stopped by on the day of admission and asked open-ended low-key background questions about her and her mother. As Wendy visited more, she recognized Jeff's skill in keeping her mother occupied and his tolerance for her mother's bizarre appearance and behavior. The DEBUT group gave her concrete information about nursing home schedules and environment. With DEBUT support, she took her idea for a fenced-in outdoor area to the administrator. Wendy gained insight and support from individual therapy as well. She realized that her fears for her mother were also fears for herself—"Who will be there for me if this happens to me?" Gradually, little incidents like her mother's inability to help with baking force Wendy to accept the terminal nature of her mother's illness despite its up-and-down course. Once she accepted her mother's terminal condition, she could plan for what she would do when "all the running stopped."

Emily and Wendy's stories illustrate the loneliness of terminal care decisions for a demented parent. Daughters are faced with decisions regarding equally unattractive alternatives—turning their homes into nursing centers without institutional economies of scale or turning their parents over to strangers. Feelings of failure, guilt, ambivalence, and prolonged grief are inevitably built into such no-win situations. In the best of all possible worlds, parents wouldn't have to experience this devastating loss of adult capacity, and daughters wouldn't have to watch helplessly.

Professionals learn that family conflict often intensifies with terminal care decisions. Again, family members may view options differently based on their past and current relationship with the parent and their understanding of the condition. Family values may dictate preferences, but all family members may not subscribe to the same values. Each may have competing commitments, and often preferred care options like live-in help aren't available, affordable, or dependable. While money increases one's options, children and parents may feel differently about the use of available assets for long-term care. Some regions of this country don't have enough nursing homes, and many don't have the intensity or skilled level of home health services required.

Wise daughters seek the support of the parent's physician. A physician's referral is required for placement, and a trusted professional can validate that the family has indeed done all that is reasonable. A family conference with help from a trusted health or social service professional is the next important step. All members of the family should be included. Those family members not invited can sabotage the placement at a later date. The conference offers time for all members to air preferences, needs, priorities, and conflicting commitments.

A skilled professional can often help a family to recognize both potential losses and gains with institutional care.

Support groups offer excellent checklists and guidelines for families to use in evaluating available services and facilities. A wise professional will help a daughter recognize that the best place for her parent is often the most convenient place for the most important family visitors. Patients with interested, consistent family visitors always get better care. Sometimes, the best place is wherever your trusted family physician visits regularly. The physician who knows you and your family over time can be invaluable in late care support and decision-making.

After a location is selected, the single most important variable is consumer recommendations. Support groups can link a daughter with other families of dementia patients in a given facility. The quality of care in any facility is determined by the hands-on personnel and the administration. Both groups experience high turnover, so it is important to talk with families of *current* residents. Visit a prospective facility for a scheduled tour to have your checklist questions answered first. Then try to visit two more times unannounced during meals, on a weekend, or at night. Observe the interaction among staff and residents, and how much help is available to those who can't feed themselves. The quality of interaction among residents, visitors, and staff is a much better criteria for dementia patients than a silent, sterile, hospital-like environment. Other regular visitors and the more intact other residents may become important supports for daughters visiting parents who are unable to communicate.

A second family conference is often precipitated as deterioration accelerates after placement. It's helpful to begin discussing the ethical "what-ifs" of care with the physician and other family members before a crisis develops. Be sure you are clear on the physician's *and* the facility's philosophy and practice on issues of feeding, treatment of infections, and hospitalization. This second family conference is an excellent opportunity to clarify terms which may be familiar only to health professionals. Daughters need clear information on the alternatives—what types of feeding tubes or hydration are possible, and what are the anticipated risks or outcomes with these procedures? Will family conflict intensify with the consequences of our choices? The tough issues for families facing terminal dementia care are *not* issues of high-tech life support. They are the more difficult issues of feeding, hydration, treatment of recurrent infections, or aggressive treatment of other unrelated but potentially fatal illnesses. Most daughters opt for comfort, meaning good nursing care, as managing nutrition, incontinence, and skin breakdown becomes most salient. Despite all this, many daughters are surprised by their unanticipated reluctance to let go. They may say in advance, "no tubes," but change their minds as the situation changes.

The final terminal care decision for families of dementia patients is a decision about autopsy. A diagnosis of Alzheimer's can only be confirmed upon autopsy. Many families also recognize the value of clinically well-documented brain tissue for genetics research. Unfortunately, it is difficult to arrange for autopsy without professional assistance. ADRDA chapters offer information and assistance with diagnostic autopsies, and Alzheimer's research centers can arrange tissue donations for research. If a decision for an autopsy will irreparably mar future family relationships, it probably isn't worth it. But many families are reluctant to permit autopsy because they don't understand what is involved and how it may affect future generations.

Daughters also have special needs during the terminal phase of a parent's illness. Just after placement, many daughters are temporarily disoriented by the new unfilled time. They find themselves equally uncomfortable at the nursing home or at home worrying about what is happening in their absence. It takes time to reorient and reschedule a more meaningful daily life. Separation after years of constant care is also difficult. Daughters frequently awaken to nightmares in which their parents are calling out to them. They need help from support groups, family, friends, and professionals in facing a future without a beloved parent.

Many daughters are surprised by their need for altruistic outlets. They realize that even the best care won't save their parent, but maybe they can do something to help others facing similar losses. This is often the time when daughters first turn to ADRDA support groups. They may be surprised to learn that they can help and be helped simultaneously. They take comfort in a shared loss and build confidence and competence in reviewing their genuinely heroic responses to difficult, no-win situations. Some daughters become active lobbyists for change or research, and others share their insights using previously untapped talents for writing, speaking, or art. Their outreach to others becomes a legacy and a way to honor the parent's memory. They try to summarize in a meaningful way what was done and why. "My five years of care for mother were not in vain—I helped others recognize they are not alone or crazy for feeling as they do, and my children better appreciate our family solidarity."

> He ladles the flaming brandy with flair. . . . He winks and you both laugh. But the dream fizzles and dies. He's far away. Your grandmother sits by his side. Your mom watches her father's flaming spirit fade. And you. You make a life. You go on. And the guilt burns. Because you're not there. Yet, if you leave your hearth to sit by his, what then? Both fires will surely die. . . . Instead, you must take up the ladle and flame the brandy. The torch is being passed. Take up the torch.—Susan Burney (ADRDA Eastern North Carolina; January 1987)

FINAL THOUGHTS

If you are fortunate, you and your family will have time to say good-bye, to reminisce, to find your own meaning in the experience, and to face the future unafraid. One daughter looked back on her mother's illness, and offered this advice for coping with "the long good-bye":

If your loved one is in the early stages, savor your conversations, and let her reminisce. . . . You will cherish those times in the days ahead.

If you are struggling through the middle stages, listen to those you love, and if they tell you to give up your loved one to professional care, give it serious thought. Children should not have to lose both parents.

And if you are in the final stages of this devastating illness, take solace that when it is over, it becomes possible to remember her as she was before, and the good memories are a great and unexpected gift.

Sheila Kane King (Des Moines,
Iowa ADRDA, 1986)

REFERENCES AND SUGGESTED READINGS

GENERAL

Advice for Adults with Aging Parents or a Dependent Spouse. Newsletter, 1985. Available from Helpful Publications, Inc., 310 W. Durham St., Philadelphia, PA 19119-2901.

Andrus Volunteers. *Who Cares? Helpful Hints for Those Who Care for a Dependent Older Person at Home*. Los Angeles: Andrus Gerontology Center, University of Southern California, 1985.

Brody, Elaine. "Parent Care as a Normative Family Stress." *The Gerontologist* 25, no. 1 (1985):19–29. Article summarizes current research and theory on family care issues.

Change. Newsletter of the National Support Center for Families of the Aging. P.O. Box 245, Swarthmore, PA, 19081. For middle generation adults facing a variety of social/health/financial dilemmas with aging parents.

George, L. K. "The Burden of Caregiving," *Center Reports on Advances in Research* 8, no. 2 (1984). Duke University Center for the Study of Aging and Human Development, Box 2920 Duke Medical Center, Durham, NC 27710.

Hooyman, N.M. and W. Lustbader. *Taking Care: Supporting Older People and Their Families*. New York: Free Press, 1986.

Kushner, Harold. *When Bad Things Happen to Good People*. New York: Schocken Books, 1982.

Manning, Doug. *When Love Gets Tough: The Nursing Home Decision*. Hereford, TX: In-Sight Books, 1985. A minister reflects on his decision to place his mother in a nursing home.

Nassif, Joan. *The Home Health Care Solution*. New York: Harper and Row, 1985.

Newsweek. "Who's Taking Care of Our Parents?" May 6, 1985.

Parent Care: Resources to Assist Family Caregivers. Newsletter. Gerontology Center, 316 Strong Hall, The University of Kansas, Lawrence, KS 66045. Rural focus.

Richards, Marty. *Choosing a Nursing Home: A Guidebook for Families.* Seatlle: University of Washington Press, 1985.

Silverstone, Barbara and Helen Hyman. *You and Your Aging Parent.* 1982. Best general reading on feelings as well as how to look for help.

SPECIFIC

Cohen, D. and C. Eisdorfer. *The Loss of Self: A Family Resource for the Care of Alzheimer's Disease and Related Disorders.* New York: Norton, 1986.

Coping and Caring: Living with Alzheimer's Disease. Washington, DC: AARP, 1986. Free from Fulfillment, 1909 K Street NW, Washington, DC 20049.

Duke Alzheimer's Family Support Program. Box 2914. Duke Medical Center, Durham, NC 27710. (919) 684-2328 and in North Carolina (800) 672-4213. A North Carolina central information point for families and professionals caring for memory-impaired elders. Complimentary general and specific information packets sent upon request; newsletter, *The Caregiver,* published quarterly; linkage to chapters and support groups of ADRDA (Alzheimer's Disease and Related Disorders Association); manuals for support group organizers; and a telephone hotline for questions, diagnosis, and management of memory disorders.

Gwyther, Lisa P. *Care of Alzheimer's Patients.* 1985. Published by ADRDA and the American Health Care Association for nursing home staff and families coping with behavior and communication problems in dementia patients. Available from ADRDA chapters or Duke Alzheimer's Program. In North Carolina call 1-800-672-4213.

HIP Report. *Help for Incontinent People.* Newsletter. P.O. Box 544, Union, SC 29379.

Levine, Susan. *Coping with Parkinson's Disease.* 1986. Free manual. The American Parkinson Disease Association, Washington University School of Medicine, Box 8111, 660 S. Euclid, St. Louis, MO 63110.

Lunt, Susan. *A Handbook for the Disabled: Ideas and Inventions for Easier Living.* New York: Charles Scribners & Sons, 1982.

Mace, Nancy L. and Peter V. Rabins. *The 36-Hour Day.* Baltimore: The Johns Hopkins University Press, 1981. Best guide to coping with early Alzheimer's Disease and other memory disorders. Available from ADRDA chapters.

Noyes, Lin E. *What's Wrong with My Grandma?* 1982. Book for small children explaining Alzheimer's Disease. Available from ADRDA-Northern Virginia, 200 East Broad Street, #1, Falls Church, VA 20046.

OWL OBSERVER. Newsletter of the Older Women's League, 1325 G Street NW, Lower Level B, Washington, DC 20005. Helpful consumer information for caregivers, homemakers and single older women.

Willing, Jules. *The Reality of Retirement.* New York: William Morrow, 1981. Inner feelings associated with white middle class retirement as a couple or family.

WHAT ABOUT SONS?

Throughout this book the role of women as caregivers for older persons has been preeminent. There is no doubt that women are actively seeking to clarify their roles and responsibilities in uncharted territory. We should not lose sight of the fact, however, that caregiving happens in a family *system*. One person assuming a task may mean that another person doesn't. Hence, we have to ask, "What about the men in this family?" This chapter tries to address that question.

In his family scenario, Michael provides us with a frank and compelling picture of one man's introduction to hands-on caregiving and his evolution in that role. He represents, we believe, a model which should be emulated, and, we discover, *a man can indeed do it!*

Writing as an anthropologist and speaking to men, not women, Phil suggests that greater empathy for caregivers can be achieved if one understands the historical roots of received attitudes and values and if one sees the connection between specific caregiving behaviors and strongly held personal beliefs about family, old age, and gender identity. He reminds us, however, that beliefs and values can change over time and that there is no good biological reason for letting men off the hook as potential caregivers.

A Son's Viewpoint
Michael Klaybor

This description of my family, my feelings, and my perspective on myself as a caregiver has been developed with the advantages of hindsight, five years of memories, psychotherapy, conversations with my wife Gayle, and input from friends and other family members. I chose to confront my feelings—and fears about my own mortality and grief—in order to deal with all of the issues involved in gaining some understanding about life, death, and parental influence. I am sharing with readers in the hope that my experience may serve to sensitize them to ways of dealing appropriately and effectively with feelings and the caregiving role in a way that preserves self-respect, independence, and dignity for everyone involved.

In the Klaybor family, we learned how to be caregivers at a very early age. By the times I was eleven, I had experienced the death of all four of my grandparents. My parents were very involved in several aspects of their care, especially after my two grandmothers died. The ideal of "strength" guided caregiving in my Polish-American family. Being a large and extended family helped to bolster that strength. I believe my observation of caregiving for grandparents will make for strong bonds in descending generations.

There were three boys and one girl in our immediate family: Marsha (the eldest), Michael (me), Gary, and Kevin. Jerry (our half-brother) was about fifteen years older and not in our immediate family but was a significant part of our support system. In addition, my father had four sisters and one brother. Mom had three brothers and one sister. We have an extended family reaching into the hundreds, and most still reside in northern Indiana. Our roots go back one hundred years in the area, so we have developed quite an extensive and valued heritage.

During the late 1950s and early 1960s, my parents were responsible for many aspects of their parents' care. They delivered meals, did shopping, helped with

173

house and yard work, managed finances, and did whatever was necessary to prolong their parents' independence. Several family members pitched in with these activities, although Dad seemed to be ultimately responsible. This period provided a lesson in values for me with an emphasis upon respect for one's parents. Dad did whatever he could to make his parents or Mom's parents as comfortable as possible.

As I looked back to the circumstances of my father's illness and death in 1968, I became aware of the many parallels between us as caregivers. As Dad became the primary caregiver for his parents, so did I for him at the onset of his troubles. For us both, there was no question as to *whether,* but only *when and how* to help.

My mom had been quite dependent on Dad and was comfortable with that arrangement. She had never learned to drive, had stopped working for wages twenty years previously, and left all family business to Dad. Hence, Dad's illness was made especially difficult for her, and she turned to me as the source of support. During Dad's year-long hospitalization with bladder cancer, I became the responsible decision-maker in the family. The relationship between Mom and Dad was still my model, however, and I simply stepped in and did things I thought my dad would do for Mom and the family. At age seventeen, I felt proud and honored to be in this position. While everyone pitched in and took some responsibility, I seemed to take over for Dad.

Dad's bladder cancer led to a slow and difficult death. Yet he died without much warning, leaving us in shock when he simply stopped breathing. I was emotionally unprepared and felt regret about conversations we never had— conversations about his successes, his failures, and most importantly, our relationship. At that time I was afraid to talk about death and avoided confronting my own feelings and fears about a future without him.

Later, I became aware of my *anger*—anger at him for abandoning us at such a difficult time, anger at being left with little support save my position on the railroad and Dad's $47.50 per month pension. I felt anger also at medical people for not helping us prepare for his death. I decided not to let that happen again and vowed to take more responsibility and ask more questions. I would acknowledge my own feelings of helplessness the next time. Despite anger directed toward the medical staff, I realized I had been deceiving myself also, and found it easy to put off taking care of important emotional business.

Dad's dying was a difficult and painful experience for us all. The event of his death marked my formal ascension to his role as the family leader. Mom gave me Dad's diamond ring and I wore it on my left hand, third finger, not thinking at the time about the symbolic significance of that gesture. Again I stepped into a role without much thought of consequences, gains, or losses—I created an entirely new life for myself overnight. I postponed college without hesitancy for it seemed impossible for me to leave at such a difficult emotional time. I was Mom's new support, and the entire family needed help to stay intact. We had extensive medical bills, no savings, and a pension that paid only half of the monthly mortage. Moreover, I discovered that Mom was now a patient too.

Soon after Dad's death, Mom's health began failing in many ways. She had an anemic collapse from being so rundown and drained from Dad's illness, trips to the hospital, and the funeral. We discovered that Mom had high blood pressure, diabetes, glaucoma, and was otherwise totally depleted.

This time around, taking care of the family meant learning as much as I could about financial assistance programs—V.A., food stamps, Social Security, housing allowances, and so forth—most of which seemed just beyond our grasp given our "lower middle" income status. Eventually, we got enough assistance to make ends meet, but the effort required a tremendous amount of patience and humility. With my work (eighty to ninety hours a week at times), my brother Gary's new salary (he turned eighteen and got a job), and Dad's veteran's benefits, we pulled through. Marsha was now setting up a family of her own, and Kevin was sixteen.

Having managed to take some course work at our local university branch campus, I felt as if my own life did have some direction. Yet, when it came time to leave home to attend the main campus, I was both excited and scared. With Gary and Kevin working and with Marsha around to help Mom, it seemed possible to leave. Mom's advanced arteriosclerotic condition, however, did cause her continuing pain, fatigue, and lack of mobility.

I became a commuter caregiver for the next three years. Mom underwent four by-pass operations: two in her legs and two heart by-passes. She slowly recovered but received little relief from numbness and pain in her legs and feet. Mom became more dependent on pain medications and took other medications for high blood pressure and glaucoma. She wasn't sleeping or eating properly either. As for me . . . I came home on weekends to take care of family business and work on the railroad.

After three years of commuter caregiving, I completed my master's degree, having switched from foreign languages to counseling. Again I returned home to take up residence with Mom, and she was delighted when I landed a good job in South Bend as director of Special Student Services.

I felt comfortable with the idea of continuing as primary caregiver while being able to start my own professional career. Our two-story home proved inconvenient so we purchased a one-story home and, for the next four years, lived rather comfortably and easily, despite Mom's deteriorating condition.

Mom's pain, however, was unrelenting. While we were financially more secure, my role as caregiver became increasingly distressing. Mom sought escape from her pain, and I began to seek escape from my role and responsibility as primary caregiver. I was beginning to feel more helpless, more angry, and more resentful toward her for being sick. Yet, my sense of obligation kept these feelings repressed. Being her favorite son and helper, how could I tell her my feelings?

Resentment grew also at being trapped and restricted in my private life. Living at home made sexuality difficult. Even the thought of emotional involvement with a woman was overwhelming, since I was already so enmeshed. As a coping strategy, I kept very busy, avoided intimacy, and sought out only very strong, independent, and active women. I realize now that many of these things were happening at a level outside my awareness.

Directing my energy toward work gave me a good excuse to partially detach from the caregiving role, and, ironically, I became quite a champion for handicapped students at the university. I was finding that my own counseling skills and compassion for others were growing. I designed special programs for handicapped students and authored accessibility studies; I even became a member of a national task force on the handicapped. In retrospect, I find that my involvement with Mom's disabilities and dependence increased my sensitivity to others and that I hadn't detached myself from a caregiving role as much as I had thought.

In 1976, I made an important decision to return to the main campus to complete a doctorate in counseling and psychology. Feeling trapped by my job—and by Mom—I needed to break away. At the same time, I became aware of and worried about *my own* dependency. I felt I needed to deepen my life outside of the comfort and security of living at home and taking care of Mom. Mom herself was deeply upset and scared about my leaving since I had been her basic support for the previous four years, indeed, since Dad's death. Hence, leaving created both a great sense of guilt and a real sense of freedom.

Mom's health at this time continued to deteriorate. An appointment with an orthopedic surgeon was necessary due to spreading gangrene—an infection that was slowly taking advantage of her poor peripheral circulation. Bravely, Mom agreed to amputations. Not wanting a complete amputation, she endured three partial amputations in the course of one year—toes, then foot, and finally, the leg to her knee.

Fortuitously, my plan to leave the scene required that Mom's other children cooperate to arrange for her care, and thus my brothers and sisters had a greater opportunity to help. Indeed, Marsha took Mom into her own home temporarily after each surgery, and this was of immense importance. The wounds required daily bandage changes, cleaning, and frequent visits to the doctor. Yet, despite our successes in "taking care of business," I regret that Marsha and I didn't get together to discuss our feelings. We worked, instead, to maintain a cheerful attitude and never shared the sadness, the fears, the pain, and the stresses we felt as a result of Mom's problems.

Mom, also, was turning inward. Not wanting to be such a burden, she was keeping her feelings to herself as we did. I exhorted her to try an artificial leg, and she finally relented but never mastered its use. As she lost weight and became weaker, the wooden leg became a barrier, not an aid, to her independence. Additionally, she was having difficulty accepting her body image changes. That summer spent at home with Mom, prior to the fall semester, was a tortuous period. I felt bound to help Mom set new goals with her body and constantly felt uncertain regarding how much I should push her to improve. Her depression pulled her backward, so I became more zealous in response. I was becoming calloused living with this on a day-to-day basis, and, looking back, I feel my strategy should have been one of encouragement with sensitivity and compassion. Indeed, it is hindsight that informs me of her bravery and endurance. The bi-weekly visits to the doctor linger vividly in my mind. The doctor would have to debride her wound without anesthetic (remove dead tissue from around the amputation). Holding my hand as the doctor worked, she would squeeze tightly, never uttering a sound, as the tears rolled down her cheecks.

The pain of Mom's leg that summer affected me in another way. I had become involved in karate as a way to release pent-up frustrations, and that summer I developed problems in my own left ankle. These chronic sprains and pains were to last another five years, only to disappear with Mom's death—a fact I realized only later.

We did, however, make it through the summer. Perhaps it was my sense of relief at being away that left me totally unprepared for the feelings that followed once I arrived on campus. Almost immediately I felt overwhelmed by all of my own changes, classes, the long ordeal of the doctorate, and leaving Mom. I was full of unresolved feelings and pent-up emotions—scared of the loss of security and control I had as a caregiver. Entering psychotherapy for the first time, I began a process of thinking and sorting out my feelings of anger, sadness, and grief. A loving guide by the name of Austin Parker assisted me as a wellspring of emotions came bursting forth. He knew how to support me and gave me permission to explore this dark and forbidding territory of my emotions. In time I came to accept myself and forgive my parents for their mortality, and began to chart a new course for my emotional growth. It prepared me to deal with my mother's impending death and opened me to the possibility of forming some deep and meaningful relationships with women. I met Gayle, my future wife, who helped me face myself and helped me move my dad's ring from my left hand to my right.

As I charted my new life, Mom became closer to Marsha, her own sister Alice, neighbors, and other relatives. With me away, there was more room for other people to share in her care. Her health, nonetheless, declined and I was away at school when the problems with gangrene developed in her other leg. Once, while I was visiting, she made a prophetic announcement that if she were to lose her right leg, she did not want to continue living. One year later that decision became a reality.

We had known that more operations might be necessary but still felt shock with the gravity of the situation. Mom was to have her entire leg removed at the hip. We were losing Mom piece by piece, and with Mom, we had an ever-increasing sense of depression and loss. Perhaps it was comic relief that caused me to spontaneously shout, upon entering her hospital room, "I forgot to put on my deodorant today!" Whatever, our collective sense of doom was temporarily displaced by laughter that day of her operation.

Mom spent several weeks in the hospital and eventually recovered enough to be released to convalesce at Marsha's house. Planning a visit home one weekend I called Marsha only to find Mom sleeping. I told Marsha I would plan a surprise visit to cheer Mom up and would use some hypnosis to help her with pain control as we had done in the past. On Friday of that week, Marsha called me back— Mom had died of heart failure. My first reaction was to remember Mom's statement about not wanting to live legless. Her prophecy had come true.

My grief over Mom's death was unlike that I experienced with my dad. The call from Marsha was a shock, yet I was prepared for Mom's death. The difference was one of communication. Regretting unspoken conversations with my dad about his life and death, I strove to share openly with Mom regarding her ordeal during that last year. Consequently, my grieving process was much shorter, cleaner, and easier.

My life as a favorite son, caregiver, surrogate husband, brother, and person has been dramatically influenced by my relationship with my parents, especially Mom. I now live a deeper, more meaningful, compassionate, empathetic, expressive life with Gayle, my children, and my close friends. My professional life was shaped by my life experiences. They led me on a journey from plans for being a high school teacher and coach like my brother, Jerry, to becoming a psychotherapist, hypnotist, geriatric specialist, and crisis worker. My goal was to gain self-knowledge to help myself and in so doing be a better guide to others. The richness of all of my experiences has uncovered my love of teaching and sharing through communication, something we didn't do enough of at home.

My parents cared for their parents and did what they could. Feeling inadequate to handle all of the feelings and experiences, I chose to go to the heart of my fears and learn about death and dying through many channels including: conducting support groups for cancer patients, specializing in treating pain of all sorts, working with families of cancer patients, and trying to help people understand their feelings. It has been an on-going experience to handle the joys and regrets associated with my parents. I still get a little uptight when Gayle, Arielle, or Adam get sick. Pain and suffering are difficult to handle, and I sometimes withdraw when I feel helpless.

Forgiveness and acceptance are the two biggest helpers I have found in my own search for inner peace. I was a significant force in my mother's life and couldn't imagine doing anything differently.

This story does not reflect the numerous contributions Gary, Kevin, Jerry, Marsha, Alice, and others made during Mom's illness. I feel the family contribution encompasses an attitude I saw reflected throughout Mom's and Dad's families as they cared for their parents. It seems this bonding and support are the most important things a family can offer and share.

Caregiving and Men's Issues
Philip B. Stafford

To the Daughters . . .

I struggled with this chapter. I found it difficult to decide *who* to talk to about men's caregiving issues. Talking to daughters regarding what they should do about their husbands and brothers seemed inappropriate—another burden for change put on the daughters' shoulders.

Hence, I've written to the men. *Don't read this chapter yourself.* Pass it along to your husband, your brother, or other men you'd like to get involved in this business of caregiving.

To the Son or Husband . . .

Dear John, or Jim, or Joe,

She's done it. She's given this to you to read. Why? you ask. Why is she so wrapped up and emotional about this whole thing? She spends twenty hours a week on top of her job to take care of her mother. You tell her to do less and she says, how? Yet, the more she does the more her mother wants. You offer to do more from time to time, and she says she's the only one who knows how to do it. The more she does the less satisfied she is. She blames you. You can feel it. You're not feeling, she says. If you have to ask what to do, don't bother, she says. You're beginning to hate Mother for what she's doing to your lover. You're angry with your lover for constantly giving in to Mother's demands. Stand up to her! you say. Hire someone to help! you say. . . .

How, you ask, did all this happen? What can I do to really help?

Well, it's a long story.

Philip Stafford, PhD, practices and teaches anthropology in Bloomington, Indiana. His interest in "old stuff" is long-standing and pervasive—ranging from old people to old songs to old houses. With his wife, Linda, and two daughters, he has settled near the old people in his family.

You see, it all started when somebody, somewhere, decided that men were more valuable than women. How this happened, I can't tell you. No one really knows, but it happened a few hundred centuries ago. Despite the fact that men were hunters, in reality women secured most of the protein for the tribe. While a man had an obvious and necessary role at conception, women really carried the children into adulthood. Despite the fact that men seemed physically stronger, it was the women who had the endurance for the long run into old age.

Nevertheless, despite your natural inferiority to women, you were the desired child. When you were born, you were accepted—the fair-haired boy. You could get away with a lot. You could be aggressive because you were "all boy." You could get away with things because "boys will be boys."

Your wife and your sister, on the other hand, didn't quite have it the same. Their female ancestors were a disappointment to their parents. Many of them were killed at birth because they weren't boys (and so didn't get a chance to be your ancestor, did they?). Your sister past had to struggle for her acceptance. She didn't automatically inherit. She didn't get the whole farm, only a dowry (which went to her husband or father-in-law). She didn't get the college tuition—that went to her brothers. She didn't get the same salary if she worked outside the home. In short, she didn't get a lot of things because she was female, not the least of which was unconditional acceptance by her parents.

When you are the recipient of automatic, unconditional acceptance, what kind of a person will you be? Well, you *won't* be overly concerned about what people think of you. You won't be very sensitive to other's thoughts and feelings. You won't be a perfectionist because you know if you don't meet a standard, you'll still be loved. Now, you might be worried about these things in areas of life outside of the family. You might worry about what your boss thinks, how your lawn looks to the neighbors, and things like that. You see, these are areas where you're *supposed* to be sensitive as a man. In fact, you get embarrassed when your wife mows the lawn or drives you in the car because people might think you're not a real man. In fact, you shy away from women's things to maintain that sense of manness. What women's things, you say? Why, things like cooking and housecleaning and lingerie departments and driving your elderly mother to the doctor. It's not that you wouldn't really *want* to do these things. In fact, there are some ways you can get around it—ways you can do domestic things and still be a man. You can cook outside like the ancient hunter in the wild. You can clean the things that are men's things—the garage, the car, the driveway. You can be around women's lingerie if you're being helped privately by a nice, plump, postmenopausal saleslady. You can even drive your elderly mother to the doctor, or the grocery store, or the pharmacy. What? I can? you say. How can I do *that* and feel rignt? How can I be her helper—do this "domestic" thing—and still be a man?

Well, first read about Michael (in "A Son's Viewpoint"). There you'll see what it is possible to do. Then, try to imagine what your wife or sister is going through. Don't ask her to feel less—you try to feel more. Don't tell her to do less because perhaps she can't. You see, she's not only trying to help, she's trying to please. She's not only being a caregiver, she's trying to be a daughter. She's trying to achieve a standard when standards of perfection in this work don't even exist yet. You can't help more because you're already acceptable in your parents' eyes. You can't do more because *you* can't be a daughter.

Is there no way out of this dilemma, you ask? There is, I think, or at least to some extent. The trick is in knowing some things you can do to get through this as an intact couple:

> Don't ask where you can help. Look for the opportunity, seize it, and don't ask for your wife's thanks when you're done. You're not simply doing it for her, you're a child of the parent too. Try on some "feminine pursuits." I don't mean that you should go out and try on your wife's underwear. I mean learn to cook a casserole. If you can't take on the behavior yet, just imagine yourself cleaning the bathroom bowl, talking all by yourself to your child's teacher, bathing your parent's naked body. Does this seem rough? Well, it is . . . and it's something that women expect to do.

Now your wife might not just let all this happen. You see, when you do something in her bailiwick, she too might feel threatened or embarrassed. So don't wait for the invitation because it may not come. She may think that you really *can't* do these things because you're a man.

Be your wife's companion. Realize that successful marriages throughout history have been based on a division of labor. It's often okay for women to do women's things and men to do men's things, and this may have been true of your marriage all along. This balance can still work for you now. Just remember that if she's a wage earner, she's already doing a "man's thing," and so you need to reciprocate. Keep it fair. You both have only twenty-four hours in a day.

More than anything else, your wife needs a friend. If she takes on too much, tell her you're concerned and realize how hard it is to do less. If she's trying too hard to please as a daughter, then see that she gets some recognition from her (your) parents, her peers, her (your) children.

ADDENDUM

Whether you're a daughter who couldn't resist reading this chapter or a son or husband, I hope you'll forgive my tendency to stretch the messages a bit. Perhaps I've been too condescending toward men. My goal is not to continue the battle of the sexes, but to promote mutual understanding and empathy.

Reading about Michael's role as a caregiver should reaffirm the belief that men are perfectly capable of being nurturant, of feeling guilt, and of performing the "bed and body work." Michael and other men caregivers seem to experience the same dilemmas, share the same pains, and achieve the same sense of satisfaction as women.

Surely much of the knowledge of caregiving has been carried on through women's oral tradition, and men perhaps have been at a disadvantage in being left out of the conversation. Women's "domestic victories," likewise, have not received their due recognition. History is too often written as the story of great *men*. The lack of press, however, in no way diminishes the value of those millions of women who have carried family life through struggle and loss.

Few modern couples exemplify roles characteristic of hunter-gatherer societies. Yet, none of us are so liberated that gender no longer means anything in our relationships. Traditions die hard, and there's a reason for this. Traditions help give meaning to our lives. They are the basic substance for sculpting our notions of self, of interpersonal relations, of right and wrong. Indeed, traditions don't die. We are never free of culture, our way of looking at the world. That's what distinguishes us from our fellow animals.

At the same time, traditions aren't handed to us ready-made. A good part of the distress we all feel, society-wide, has to do with the fact that new standards and ethics of caregiving are only dimly perceived. Today's daughters are cultural trailblazers. The maps they create, describing the new caregiving roles, will be the next generation's traditions. Men need not miss the wagon in this venture. As men discover the joys of child rearing, so can they help discover the pains *and* satisfactions of caregiving for their elderly parents.

A Note on Research: Men as Caregivers

Within recent years, many researchers have begun examining the character and scope of caregiving in families with dependent elders. Perhaps our greatest depth of gratitude should be extended to Ethel Shanas and her coworkers at the University of Chicago. Her nationwide and cross-national surveys in the late sixties utilizing large samples of respondents, documents without a doubt, that *most* caregiving for dependent elderly is done by family members, not health care professionals (Shanas 1968, 1979a, 1979b). The myth that families give up on their elderly relatives who are ill has been effectively debunked, though it occasionally rears its head.

Through the excellent and durable research efforts of Elaine Brody and colleagues at the Philadelphia Geriatric Center, another "truth" about caregiving has been revealed. In many studies, she has documented that caregiving is primarily the work of women. Brody's graphic picture of the "woman in the middle" is now a standby (Brody 1981).

Other, more recent, surveys on larger samples of caregivers bear out the original theme. Amy Horowitz, through studies conducted at the Brookdale Center on Aging, (1985) surveyed a sample of 288 elderly and 203 caregivers in New York City. In her sample "seventy percent of all adult children originally identified as primary caregivers by their parents were female" (1985, 614). Most males who were primary caregivers tended to be such by virtue of a demographic reality (only child, adult children in male-only sibling networks, or the only child in the geographic area).

One of the most extensive surveys of caregiving patterns was completed by the National Center for Health Services Research on a national sample (Stone and Cafferata 1986). Stone and Cafferata found that in their sample, 29 percent of the primary caregivers were adult daughters, 23 percent were wives, and only 13 percent were husbands. (Of course, the age differential in marriages of our current elderly means that most wives have older husbands and the men are likely to fall ill first.)

Colleen Johnson (1983), has described a principle of "substitution" at work in many families. If the spouse of a dependent elder is alive, that person usually becomes the primary caregiver. (The spouse is usually female.) If no spouse is alive or able, caregiving responsibilities fall upon an adult child. (The adult child "nominated" is usually a female.) If no women are around, men pick up the reins. If both men and women are available, then women usually do more and provide most of the instrumental assistance with activities of daily living. Men typically assume a more distant role as financial advisors or decision-makers.

As many writers have pointed out, despite the increasing participation of women in the work force (especially middle-aged women), there has not been a decline in the amount of caregiving hours provided to dependent elders by daughters. Most women will either cut back the number of hours on their jobs (or quit altogether), or simply add the ten, fifteen, or twenty weekly caregiving hours to their already full-time job.

An interesting finding of the Horowitz study indicates that male caregivers seem to experience less stress in the caregiving role (when level of involvement is controlled for in the study). It is hypothesized that men have less of an emotional involvement in the intimacies of caregiving, though at present, this is merely speculative. Perhaps the tendency of men to underrepresent their true feelings produced an artifact in the research. It would be worthwhile to examine the long-range consequences of exhausting caregiving with this gender issue in mind.

In summary, it's safe to agree that parent care is, in our society, a women's issue. One shouldn't agree, however, that that's the way it *has* to be. If men experience less stress, then perhaps they have some things to teach women about caregiving. At the same time, women have a world of experience as nurturant caregivers, which can and should be shared with men. If a total exchange of roles is *not* possible, then certainly a complementary, partnership approach to caregiving *is*.

REFERENCES

Brody, Elaine. " 'Women in the Middle' and Family Help to Older People," *The Gerontologist* 21(1981): 471–80.

Horowitz, Amy. "Sons and Daughters as Caregivers to Older Parents: Differences in Role Performance and Consequences," *The Gerontologist* 25, no. 6 (1985): 612–17.

Johnson, Coleen. "Dyadic Social Relationships and Social Support," *The Gerontologist* 23, no. 4 (1983): 377–83.

Johnson, Coleen and D. Catalano. "Childless Elderly and Their Family Supports," *The Gerontologist* 21, no. 6 (1981): 616–18.

Shanas, Ethel (a). "Social Myth as Hypothesis: The Case of the Family Relations of Old People," *The Gerontologist* 19(1979): 3–9.

Shanas, Ethel (b). "The Family as a Social Support System in Old Age," *The Gerontologist* 19(1979): 169–74.

Shanas, Ethel et al. *Old People in Three Industrial Societies.* New York: Atherton Press, 1968.

Stone, R. and G. L. Cafferata. "Caregivers of the Frail Elderly," paper presented at American Society on Aging, cited in National Center for Health Services Research and Health Care Technology Assessment, *Research Activities,* no. 87 (July 1986).

THE LAST OF LIFE

When adult children discover that their parents may be dying, family relationships are tested, sometimes cruelly, and effective communication between caregivers and health professionals becomes even more crucial to caregiving and decision-making. Well-established, reciprocal interaction with physicians and other health care professionals can significantly ease a family's pain or burdens.

Virginia allows us to walk with her through the unexpected discovery of her mother's impending death, a series of experiences with health care providers, and her family's transitions and adjustments while providing care for her dying mother. Dr. Glen Davidson, chairman of the Department of Medical Humanities at Southern Illinois University, has experienced the loss of both his parents and now calls himself on orphan. His excellent book, *Understanding Mourning—A Guide for Those Who Grieve,* is recommended as a source of information and support for the stages of mourning.

Milton, a family practice physician, discusses the importance of partnerships that work effectively and without breakdown especially at times of crisis. He describes the Patient Advisory Council as a model to demonstrate one way of establishing a structured method for reaching agreement or compromise and resolving conflict. Tanya, an active parish priest and president of "Communicators, Inc." reminds us that throughout our life span we experience the need for forgiveness—to forgive or to be forgiven. She relates the attitudes about forgiveness to the elements and process of forgiving—forgiving ourselves as well as others.

Love Enough to Let Go

Virginia L. Marlow

In November my mother was in a small town hospital vomiting her insides out, as she had been off and on for the previous six months. According to her doctor she was having muscle spasms in her stomach. To me the doctor's usage of "muscle spasm" meant the doctor didn't know what was wrong and was too insecure to admit it. I urged my mother to come home with me and see a doctor in our medical center. She said she would, only if her doctor referred her, which he didn't. At the time, I must have been so busy in my own life that I wasn't willing to put forth the energy or the courage to challenge the diagnosis and to push for a referral. A month later, on Christmas vacation, I found my mother still in poor health. Because of this, my sister and I made an appointment to see my mother's doctor on Christmas Eve. During the visit I told him I believed something was seriously wrong with my mother; I felt that she was starving to death. She had lost forty pounds over the last several months and could keep very little food down. She had reached the point where she was afraid to eat. I told the doctor that while helping Mom change clothes the previous night, I had felt an unnatural protrusion in her stomach area. The doctor said, "You mean the muscle spasm?" However, her doctor did agree to refer Mom to a doctor at our medical center, but only after he examined her one more time.

A few days later, my sister called asking me to come, pick up Mom, and bring her to our medical center. Her family doctor had referred her to a cardiologist in our city. Mom had a heart condition, angina pectoris, and had been diagnosed four years previously as having an inoperable aneurysm. At that time her family doctor interpreted the specialist's finding as meaning that Mom would be recommended for surgery of *any kind* only as a last step. (We found out later from the cardiologist that this was not the correct interpretation.) Even with the heart condition, I was confused about the referral to a cardiologist rather than a gastrointestinal specialist. However, I was relieved by the fact that she was to be seen by a specialist, any specialist, with access to more sophisticated testing equipment.

I left home late on a Friday afternoon, arriving at Mom's that night, and the two of us headed toward our medical center the following morning. Mom traveled in her night gown and robe, propped up by pillows in the back seat of my car. We made a few "pit stops" and laughed about traveling like the Beverly Hillbillys, a joke we had shared for years. We assumed that because she was arriving at the medical center on a Saturday not much testing would be done that day. However, once Mom got checked into her room, it was like all hell tore loose. The doctor she had been referred to arrived almost immediately, examined her, said she would have a test promptly and if it showed an aneurysm on her main aorta as her family doctor suspected, she was to have emergency surgery that afternoon. I asked him to slow down. We needed time to grasp the seriousness of the situation. None of us had been informed of the possible urgency of Mom's condition. The doctor said the aorta could burst at any time, and she would die if it did so. Then he left the room.

I felt overwhelmed by emotion and a loss of control. I thought, "My God, my mom could be dead in a matter of hours. I don't know what is going on. How do I slow this process down? Once this ball gets in motion, it will be too hard to stop." I rushed out after the doctor with a feeling of helplessness and a need to see alternatives. I found the doctor at the nurses' station. I told him I needed to know more. The doctor, seemingly aggravated, began explaining the ultra-sound test. I told him I wanted to know more about the possible surgery. He said it was major, that she could die on the operating table, and that if the aneurysm burst without the surgery she would certainly die. He really told me no more than he had stated in the presence of my mother; however, I believe that I needed to have it confirmed again and have the reality of the situation filter through in order to feel I had comprehended correctly. I then told him that following the test I would need time to inform my sister of the results, and that if the operation were necessary she would need time to travel to the hospital. He asked how long it would take for her to arrive. I replied, "Three hours." He said that there would be no time to wait for her. I can remember thinking, "Mom has lived with this condition for months, now we can't wait three hours for surgery." Also, I thought, "The doctor must know what he's talking about, he's the expert, and everything must be done to save Mom."

I went back to Mom's room. We wrapped our arms around each other, and we cried. Mom said, "I'm scared. I'm not ready to die yet. I believe there are still ways in which I can contribute to life." I choked out, "I'm not ready to give you up." I remember then sitting up, blowing my nose, and saying, "Now that we've cried, Mom, it's time to get tough. I really believe you're going to make it ok. I'll give Bunny a call and tell her to come up, just in case surgery is required."

Shortly thereafter, someone came in to take Mom downstairs for the ultra-sound test. I told the lady I would ride the elevator downstairs with them. She said, "You can ride down, but they won't let you in while the testing is being done." When we met the technician, I introduced myself, acted very nice, and the technician invited me in to watch the test. (I found throughout my mom's hospital stay, that by being nice I was able to get into many places that ordinarily family couldn't go.) The technician described the different organs and said she found no aneurysm. A radiologist came in and agreed, no aneurysm, but they also agreed there was something in the stomach. About that time the surgeon who had been called for the surgery came in, watched the testing, and said to my mother, "Well, Honey, you don't need me today," and left. Needless to say we were quite relieved, and by the time my sister arrived our state of anxiety had relaxed.

The next day the testing began to find out what was causing pain in Mom's stomach. A gastrointestinal specialist and an internist were called in on Mom's case. I stayed with my mother almost constantly. She was afraid of being alone and made "no bones" about it. In the meantime, my brother in South Carolina was called and informed of Mom's condition. He and his wife decided to make the trip to see her.

After a week and a half of testing the resident who had been working with us came in and asked if any of the doctors had talked with us about their findings. We said no. (Mom and the resident had already built a warm relationship. He was raised in the same area we had come from and we had friends in common. Mom referred to him as "the doctor who speaks our language.") His eyes glazed with tears and I shall never forget his sensitivity. He described Mom's condition. There was a growth in her stomach that appeared to be malignant. The recommended treatment was the removal of half her stomach. I felt stunned, yet I remember telling my mother that she didn't have to have surgery, that it was just their recommendation, and that she had control over what was to be done to her.

Later that evening, Mom told me that since my brother, sister-in-law, and sister were arriving the next day, she wanted me to tell them *in person* of her condition before they came in to see her, but not before their arrival in town, for fear they would travel recklessly. She wanted them to deal with their pain before she saw them in order to be able to keep a positive attitude with them. She was using all her strength to maintain control of her emotions. Her role in our family had been that of a strong matriarch, and even with a tube down her throat and the intravenous needles in her arms she wasn't about to give up that position of strength.

Outstanding events that I remember from the next days are my mother's eventual consent to surgery which was changed from the removal of half her stomach to three quarter removal, telling my sister of Mom's condition, crying with her, and telling my brother and sister-in-law of Mom's condition. During all of this confusion my husband had assumed the role of primary caregiver in our home, keeping things going for our children and for everyone who was coming in and out.

Needless to say, the morning of Mom's surgery was a tense one. I can remember thinking Mom would have something profound to tell us before her surgery. (It's amazing how many assumptions we make during times of tension.) Mom's total concentration was on getting through the surgery ok. She really didn't want us to bother with her much that morning. As soon as she was taken to surgery, we went to the lounge for what we thought would be a long wait. Shortly after my husband arrived, the surgeon who had been scheduled to perform the surgery came in. As soon as I saw him, I thought, "Mom's dead!" There hadn't been time for complete surgery. The doctor told us there wasn't much they could do for Mom. The cancer was so extensive that all they did was connect her to a continuous nutritional feeding machine. While the surgeon was talking with us, I felt light-headed, as if the event wasn't real. As he talked, the only message I received was that the cancer was so extensive they could do nothing for her. I thought, "all this pain for nothing." On that day I began to mourn my mother's death. The information on the continuous feeding machine passed over the top of my head; however, it was to come back to haunt me later.

After all of us had the opportunity to go in to see Mom in the intensive care unit, my sister-in-law and I went home and rested. We then returned, prepared to spend the night. Prior to surgery, Mom had talked with the two of us and told us she thought we were the ones who would best cope with her condition following surgery. Barb and I had a plan. We decided that when we went into the intensive care unit, if we were *very quiet* and stayed out of everyone's way, the staff wouldn't notice us, and we could be allowed to stay beyond the designated five minute period. To our surprise we found the nursing staff extremely sensitive to our family situation. We didn't have to be "sneaky." The head nurse projected a great deal of empathy and understanding. She said she recognized our concern and didn't mind if we stayed as long as we wanted. All she asked was that if an emergency occurred we were to leave the area quickly and quietly.

Barb and I stood half the night holding Mom's hands. We worked out a code with Mom so she could communicate with us even with the respirator in her mouth. She spelled out words to us on our hands. After what seemed to be a long period of time we figured out the letters TOO MUCH HEAT. We then spent what seemed to be hours waving our hands back and forth across her body to create movement of air to cool her. Once we told her we were going to leave the area to get something to eat. She let us know that that would be fine, but only one at a time. I believe it relieved a great deal of Mom's fear (and ours) to be able to be with her through that first night following surgery.

At this point my sister and brother returned to their homes and jobs. My brother's wife stayed on and was extremely helpful in supporting Mom and me through each day.

Once Mom got out of intensive care, I gradually began to comprehend her situation, our situation. Throughout the ordeal, my pattern seemed to be that I was always at least one step ahead in my thinking from where the doctors wanted me to be with my questions. This created several confrontations between the doctors and me. After the surgery there gradually came to be a total of seven doctors involved in the care of my mother, and it seemed to me that each one had a different story and recommendation. "Dr. Klutz" (a title my mother had given a particular doctor because of his lack of tact) told me following some of my questions that he thought I was over-anxious and over-excited about my mother's condition. He said he had recognized this even prior to my mother's surgery. I told him if that were true, it was probably because I did not trust all doctors. He turned and walked away from me. I was furious. (Mom's past history of incorrect diagnosis fed my anxiety. I was also dealing with my anger over Mom and our family not being told that a possible outcome of the surgery was for Mom to be connected to a continuous feeding machine for the duration of her life. I felt if I didn't press with questions, the information would not be volunteered.)

I'll never forget the day "Dr. Klutz" came in and said, "We have wonderful news today. You have lymphoma rather than carcinoma. That means your cancer is treatable. We'll bring in an oncologist who will work out a plan of chemotherapy and/or radiation treatments." The idea of chemotherapy was not a pleasant prospect. Mom and I had had contact with people who had encountered such treatments. We both had heard statements like, "I would rather be dead than go through it again." We had seen people who had lost all of their hair. Mom, my sister-in-law, and I talked a great deal about the "wonderful news." While Mom was still struggling with the issue of treatment, she pinned down the resident with some pretty direct questions. I praise him for his courage to answer her questions without becoming defensive despite his discomfort, which I sensed. Mom asked him just how much the treatment would help her. He, of course, gave her information on good results, some statistics here and there as I recall. Mom pressed him further. He said there were no guarantees, but he believed treatment would prolong her life. She asked how long. His answer was vague. Then she posed the "zingers." Would the treatment cure her? He reluctantly said no. She then asked, "You mean that I could end up back in this condition again?" As I recall, he softly said, "Yes." When the resident left the room, Mom turned to me and said, "No one should go through this twice." Mother rejected chemotherapy and radiation therapy. I supported that decision. At the time I felt, from what seemed to be an angry response from several doctors, that rejection of treatment was looked upon as a stupid and unheard of decision. One doctor, while trying to convince Mom to go with the treatment, told her he had ninety-year-old patients receiving chemo treatment. In Mother's situation she would have had to have chemotherapy in conjunction with radiation for the treatment to be effective. I do not regret Mom's decision, nor do I regret supporting it.

Mom made up her mind that she wanted to be out of the hospital, and she wanted to be out right away. Then came the point of . . . ok, but what are we going to do with her? Her care was to be such that she couldn't be left alone. Her primary physician, the one who admitted her, said, "Take your mother home, don't change your life-style, and hire a nurse around the clock." I felt dumbfounded. He might as well have told me to take her to the moon. Mom was living on my deceased father's miner's pension and social security and had no assets other than her house. My husband and I are middle income people with two children in college and three at home. The family had little money for such enormous expenses. Around-the-clock nursing care cannot be done without a source of income, and that source is usually not present for most people. Later, while checking into costs, I found that Medicare doesn't cover around-the-clock in-home nursing care. A lunar trip could have been accomplished with an equal amount of ease.

As we began to think of possibilities for Mom's care, our thoughts were that she would go to her home and my sister would move back into the family household. I could go down on weekends to give her a break, and we would get some kind of outside help to stay with Mom while she worked. My sister was agreeable to the plan; yet, I knew this was not a good solution. Then we began a long round of inquiries. What kind of insurance coverage did Mom have for outside help, if any? We learned she was going to require "skilled nursing," a term I became familiar with. I began to think of my sister's social life. She was in her twenties, single, and dating was part of her life-style. How fair would this be to her? What about my sister's ability to cope with the new demands on her life? The social worker assigned to do discharge planning kept encouraging us to put Mom into a nursing home, which was out of the question . . . or was it? (I gained understanding of how people painfully reach that solution.) I came up with another plan, which was to bring Mom home to my house and have someone come in during the time I was at work and in class. Then I thought, "Well, maybe I'll quit college and hang onto my job. I can always finish school, but the money I'm making keeps the boys in college. . . . *Oh, my God, the pain of what to do . . . what to do . . . no easy answers.*"

When I talked to Mom about coming to live with us she was so receptive, so afraid, so vulnerable, so fearful of being stuck somewhere outside the family. That evening I took my husband aside, and I asked how he would feel about bringing Mom to our home to spend her remaining days with us. (Her prognosis was six months.) He asked me what I wanted. I gave a wounded cry, my knees gave away, I leaned on my husband and said, "I want her to die." (I loved her so much, yet wished her death.) We agreed to bring her to our home. I knew this wasn't a good answer; however, I felt there were no other options other than a nursing home. My stomach began to knot up, and I kept thinking, "How would it be for the three children at home to see someone they love die? Would it influence their development? How would it be for them not to have their friends in because Grandma is sick? What would it be like for them to share one bedroom? How much would they resent giving up the little privacy they had?"

By the time I got to the hospital the next day, I was a wreck. At this point

Mom had it in her head that she could leave the hospital in two days, and she had "conned" some of the doctors into agreeing. I told her she could come to our house, but that I needed more time to get myself physically and emotionally strong again. She said, "Go home and rest." I said I still needed more time to get things ready at home and to learn how to give medications through her nutritional feeding tube, empty drainage bags, and operate her machinery. She said, "You can learn it in a day." I said, "I need more time." She began to cry and shout that I was abandoning her and that she always thought I was the one person she could count on. I began to cry and said, "Mom, I have limits. I need to get myself together. I'm falling apart." She shouted, "Get out of here." I told her, "I'm not going anywhere." We had quite a scene, eventually ending up with our arms around each other crying.

By the time I got home I had rejuvenated some on the outside, for I didn't want my husband to recognize the strain of the day or how emotionally vulnerable I was becoming. When Jerry came in from work he commented on how much better I looked. I thought, "If you only knew." He told me he wanted to talk with me and that he had been thinking of Mom's situation all day. He began with, "This is only an idea for you to consider, another alternative. Realistically you know that by bringing your mom here, you're going to have to quit work and drop out of school to care for her." I nodded. He said, "I know it's important to you to be overseeing her care." I thought, how well my partner knows me, and the tears began streaming. He said, "I've been thinking about your mom and how I would feel if I were her. Your mom is coming home from the hospital to die. Why not take her where she would like to be, in the town where she has spent all her life, in her home of fifty years, where all her friends are. You can take her home, to her home. You and Bunny can help each other care for your mom. The kids and I can come down on weekends to be with you." The knot lifted from my stomach and I knew it was the answer; however, it would never have occurred to me as a solution. The knowledge of finding a right answer for all of us brought me a sense of peace I hadn't felt for five weeks. That evening I stayed away from the hospital, and we strived for a night of family normalcy. I told the children I would be leaving to take Grandma home for as long as she lived, and I didn't know just how long I would be gone. I told them their dad was going to be "Mr. Mom" and that they would be coming down to see me and their grandma every possible weekend. The kids took the news pretty well. I was the one who had a hard time keeping myself together.

The next day I told my mother of the alternate solution. I told her this would be our family gift to her. She cried and cried in thanks and praised my husband. That evening Jerry came to the hospital to see Mom. The emotions were high yet unspoken. Their eyes filled with tears. As Mom's tears began to flow she said, "Thank you for what you're doing for me." She paused, took a deep breath, wiped her tears away, and changed the subject which allowed my husband to maintain his composure.

At this point, the hospital staff seemed to think we were all completely nuts. We were now asking them to change the discharge plans for a third time. I learned that we needed time to make a major decision, to explore alternatives, and think through how the alternatives would be to live with.

In the next two days I learned how to operate the kangaroo pump, learned about irrigating the tube into her stomach, mixing and measuring nutritional feedings, administering medication through tubing, and emptying and changing the drainage bag.

In the next couple of weeks Mom and I had a few intimate exchanges, but one regret is that I didn't tell her of the emptiness I feared her loss would bring to me. I kept thinking "she needs to talk about her fears," not recognizing my need to talk with her. The sharing and reflecting upon our lives that I had hoped for never occurred. For about the first week or so we daily walked through the house, nutritional machine and all. Mom would say, "It's time to take inventory." Yet she seemed to get weaker each day. Our conversation centered around her care. In retrospect that saddens me deeply. One day she said, "All these things keep rolling around in my head." I asked her, "What kind of things?" She said, "Just things." I said, "Sometimes when we talk about things that are bothering us, they don't seem as bad." She said, "If I talk about them, they'll only be worse." One of the times that I said, "I love you, Mom," she responded, "I worship you, Virginia." I said, "Oh, Mom." Then she said, "I guess that's not right, I should only worship God." Another time she asked me how I could take care of her so willingly and cheerfully. Another time she made reference to my sister's good looks, then said, "Nobody has eyes like you."

Even though I felt terribly alone in the care and responsibility of Mother, I actually had some fantastic support. My sister and I supported each other every day. It seemed important for me to take charge, and in this particular situation, I believe she was more comfortable as support for my efforts. My sister-in-law, who had had several differences with my mother, sister, and myself over the years really came through in supporting and caring for my mother and in supporting me through extremely trying days while Mom was in the hospital. A great deal of healing took place in that relationship. My mother's adopted family (a family with whom Mom had participated in the raising of the children) were with us daily. Janie came by each evening with loving concern. Her daughter came by each noontime bringing me lunch. These people ran all over the place seeing to our comfort. "The Ladies," mother's card-playing friends also sensitively came to see Mom. Each one of them had an opportunity to be with her, express their love with understanding, and offer our family support. An RN friend who had been married to a doctor who died of cancer came by several times and checked by phone every other day. She was the only one who told me what she thought would occur at death. This helped me a great deal, for I desperately needed a mental picture so I could cope. My husband's brother took me out to dinner once, just to get me "outside the walls." This was his way of saying he cared. My husband and the children totally supported my efforts and never complained about any inconvenience resulting from my absence. My two college boys kept in contact, supporting what I was doing in the care of their grandmother. My oldest son wrote a letter to my mother with a line I shall never forget, "Grandma, I think of you each day and I smile."

Mom had chosen to continue under the care and supervision of her physician of twenty years. Initially I was very unhappy about her decision. In fact I tried to influence her into seeing a different physician; however, I respected the little control she still had over her life. Even with the incorrect diagnosis and what I saw as extreme stubbornness about making a referral, I knew he cared for her, and at that point caring for her as a person counted a lot. He came to the house twice and, basically, gave us the message we were doing everything fine. We contracted with a nursing service that was Medicare covered and had an RN come in several times a week to check blood pressure and see that all the tubing and machinery was working properly. Along with the nursing service came an aide to give baths a couple of times a week. This helped me conserve some of my strength. With all the support from family, friends, and professional caregivers, I still felt a sense of aloneness. Though my sister was frequently present, Mom became very dependent upon me. Once I internally accepted the reality of responsibility, much of my fear of making a mistake was greatly diminished.

I tried to be methodical in caring for Mom. I charted when her medications were given, the amount, her liquid intake, and the amount of discharge from her drainage bag. One of the struggles I had with Mom was over her pain medication. She never wanted to take very much, even though her discomfort was evident. I suppose she was extremely fearful her mind wouldn't be clear.

One morning my sister got up around seven to give Mom her medications. When she went to chart it she realized I had been up at five and had given some pain medication. She then came to my bedroom worried that Mom had been given too much. I told her what she had given added to what I gave still didn't exceed the limit of what a single dosage of codeine with tylenol could be.

Shortly thereafter I got up and went into Mom's room. She said she thought she had wet the bed and still felt she needed to go on the potty. (Two days prior she had fallen on the floor trying to reach the commode on her own because she did not want to disturb my sleep.) I helped her sit up. She fell backwards on the bed, and a look of disgust crossed her face. I sensed her thoughts to be, "Now I can't even sit up." I was able to get her out of bed and help her to the bedside commode, then changed the sheets and helped her get back into bed. She seemed to be resting somewhat comfortably so I said, "Mom, I'll run downstairs, get the sheets washing, and I'll be right back up." In the meantime my sister was about ready to leave for work. She went in, kissed Mom good-bye, and started out the door. I passed her on the stairs. Just as I entered Mom's room, I saw her eyes glazed over, and I screamed to my sister, "Don't leave." I knew instantly Mom was dying. I could hear her lungs filling with fluid. As my sister came to the bedroom door, I cried, "Mom's dying." Bunny went for the phone to call the ambulance. I said, *"No, I don't want her on a respirator!"* She then called the family doctor, came in, and wrapped her arms around Mom. As we both held onto Mom, I felt like we were her little children again, holding onto our life, holding onto a strength that had supported us for all our years. Yet we both knew we had to let her go on to something better than her existence had become. Even through my pain of kissing her body good-bye, I sensed her presence already outside her body watching us and loving us through our suffering. As we caressed her, verbalizing our love as our last message, she died in our arms.

Over the years since my father's death, Mom and I had had many conversations about death. She feared dying with a deteriorated mind, in a hospital away from the comfort of familiarity, as my father had. Mom had anticipated death and had shared her feelings and wishes with my sister and me. My mother knew she was dying last fall. She simply didn't know what exactly was wrong with her. She had made all funeral arrangements. She said she knew Bunny and I would be grieving so deeply for her that she would save us from those decisions. She saw it as a gift to us. On the Christmas prior to her death, as we were beginning our dinner, I said, "Shouldn't we thank God for the special gift of being together?" Mom began to cry, and the two of us left the kitchen in tears. The words were unspoken, but we knew it to be our last Christmas.

Our family received many gifts of love in our loneliness. I guess that is part of the message of my words. Other people's caring helped us make it through each day. The other part of my message is to professional caregivers. There is so much more going on throughout a medical crisis than disease and treatment. The emotional trauma should at least be acknowledged and approached with sensitivity. My mother told me once that the hardest test of my love for my children would be to love them enough to let go of them. I feel we all had the same test with my mother.

Partnerships in Health Care

Dr. Milton Seifert

Illness is inconvenient, frustrating, scary, and more costly than being well. The individual and family systems are stressed, and the flow of everyday life disturbed. The health system is necessary but it is complex enough to overwhelm any one of us. If sickness involves an elderly parent, all of these problems are multiplied. It is enough to make you want to run, but don't, because you are needed. The purpose of this chapter is to show how you can be helpful to your parent and to the health professionals and still survive the process.

The establishment of health care partnerships is a real survival skill. By connecting with resource people, health care professionals, and systems of support, you will be able to accomplish what is needed of you. The partnership style of health care is an efficient and humane way of dealing with complicated health care problems. It has led to a better definition of how doctors and patients can work collaboratively.

If you were to visit our medical practice, you would find a family physician, a physician assistant, a health educator, and the usual supporting staff. It would look usual and ordinary but we hope that the partnership concept would be evident in our attitude and our actions. One of us would tell you that our most important product is the doctor/patient relationship. We would tell you that we believe the quality of the relationship will determine the quality of the outcome of the health care services. We would let you know that the patient is as

Milton H. Seifert, Jr., MD is a family physician in general practice in Excelsior, Minnesota. He has been in full-time clinical practice since 1958 except for two years in the United States Air Force. He holds teaching appointments in family practice at the University of Minnesota and the University of Wisconsin. He has served on research committees of state, national, and international organizations. Dr. Seifert is a charter member and certified by the American Board of Family Practice. He also holds membership in the American Academy of Family Physicians, the Society of Teachers of Family Medicine, the Ambulatory Sentinel Practice Network, and the North American Primary Care Research Group.

responsible for the relationship as is the doctor. We would tell you about our health educators who teach life management skills, and we would tell you about our Patient Advisory Council where patients help other patients with health care needs or help the practice staff resolve patient complaints. You would be told that we expect to listen and to care about you and that we expect the same in return.

The partnership style is perhaps at its best in a crisis situation. It provides a way to deal with the overwhelming in a successful fashion. Things may be bad, but we feel good about what we are doing. The partnership that is best in crisis is one that is already established and has a history of successful collaboration. There is trust and a willingness to work together. In the case of an elderly parent, it is likely there has been some contingency planning for this particular crisis— you are a part of the health care team, and you are ready.

If you come to crisis without a pre-established partnership, then you put all of your energy into building a partnership because the need is still there. To be successful, you will put into your relationship-building ideas such as: cooperation, collaboration, interdependence, listening, caring, respect, appreciation, and support. It is suggested that you take your commitment to an elderly parent and use that as a power to build a health care partnership.

Knowing that you have a need for help and support is a place to begin, although it is not the first step. Having a willingness to accept help and support is also important and also not the first step. I know that you wish to provide competent care for your parents and I believe that I can help you do that. The most important thing I hope to teach you is the value of partnership health care. Sometime after I entered general practice in Excelsior, Minnesota, I began to realize that it was the patients who were teaching me how to practice medicine. In the past twenty plus years, this experience has taught me what I must do and what the patient must do, and that is what I would like to convey to you.

THE PATIENT'S ROLE IN THE PATIENT/DOCTOR RELATIONSHIP

The first step for you in helping your parents is to wear your automobile seatbelt. Why? Because that is something that you are able to do even though a lot of other things may have you feeling defeated. Partnership health care of necessity must begin with personal self-care. We all need to take care of our own health maintenance because it is not possible for someone else to do it for us. Taking the responsibility for emotional self-care makes it possible for each of us to have optimum judgment in dealing with important problems. A partnership functions best when both partners are competent and managing their own lives well. The task of caring for parents is very hard, and therefore, the caregiver must be in good health. Each of us must get into shape physically, mentally, emotionally, and spiritually. Each of us must look after our own health and strive for the greatest fitness possible. In addition to using the seatbelt, each of us should exercise every day, make a point of good nutrition, and deal with our own stresses and emotional pain. But start with your seatbelt, and when you put it on say to yourself, "This is one part of my health maintenance program. Something that is within my power. Something that I can do for myself. Let me think of the other things that I do for my own health maintenance. . . . Am I satisfied with my own health maintenance program? . . . What can I do to improve my own self-care?" So now you know the first step.

This discussion is also about the concept of managing one's own life. We all have the power to do that, you know—no matter what actual circumstances we face. We teach our patients that victimization and burn-out are self-inflicted. That may sound unfair but it isn't. Instead it gives a person the power to manage his own life regardless of the circumstances. If you believe that the circumstances are beyond your control, then they will be for sure. However, if you look at the circumstances as something within your power, then you will be able to change things.

EMOTIONAL SELF-CARE

Management of one's emotions is necessary to the self-care idea. Management of one's emotions is how we take care of our personal stresses. We teach our patients stress management skills because unmanaged feelings can distort thinking and interfere with judgment, and that is something that will interfere with both self-care and partnership functioning. We need sane thinking and good judgment when we approach any important problem. The health problems of a parent deserve our best judgment.

I will tell you some things to do in dealing with emotional pain, but first I will tell you some things not to do. Do not be a martyr. Do not be strong and silent. Do not indulge in self pity, be too independent, or think of yourself as a victim. Most of all, do not blame anybody or anything for your particular situation.

Blame is a common response to emotional pain, but it doesn't relieve pain. It is like using alcohol for emotional pain—which is also not helpful. So, the emotional pain remains but is transferred to whoever or whatever is being blamed. The unresolved pain continues to exert a negative effect on thinking and judgment. You are being victimized by your own pain, and blame puts it out of your reach. You are in fact victimizing yourself. Therefore, if you have the power to victimize yourself, you also have the power to stop victimizing yourself. You simply stop the process of blame, accept responsibility for your own pain, and then you will find you have the power to confront and deal with your emotional pain. This process is called acceptance.

In dealing with emctional pain, we ask our patients to calculate the amount of pain they feel. Then we ask them to show themselves how much it is affecting their own best judgment by completing the following exercises:

How much do I feel:

	Very low	Low	Moderate	High	Very High
Anger					
Fear					
Guilt					

What do my emotions make me feel like saying
    Anger (It makes me feel like saying):
    Fear (It makes me feel like saying):
    Guilt (It makes me feel like saying):

The above exercise allows you to detach from the things you are feeling. It lets you look at the circumstances as though you are looking at someone else. Please note how the very high emotional feelings relate to what you want to say. What you are about to say is only a step away from what you are about to do. If it looks as though you are acting in bad judgment, that would be normal with a high degree of emotional pain. If you want your own best judgment, then it is clear that you must reduce the emotional pain before you act. Management of emotional pain is the key to the obtainment of good judgment.

The following are the steps that one can take to achieve emotional self care:

    1) calculate the intensity of your emotional pain (as above)
    2) prepare for acceptance of your own emotional pain
       a) put aside blame
       b) turn the other cheek if necessary
       c) love your enemies if necessary
       d) look for the willingness to accept the ownership of your own emotional pain
    3) acceptance and ownership of your own emotional pain
    4) deal with your own emotional pain
       a) do something for yourself
       b) do something for someone else
       c) let someone help you with a personal need
       d) ask another person to help you with a personal need
       e) appreciate: people, family, places, things, and yourself

Acceptance is perhaps the most critical element in the self-management of emotional pain. When the actual facts lead easily to blame it is hard to give it up—but you can't help yourself unless you do. You can't blame anything, not even yourself. When the object of your blame is a powerful force then it may require turning the other cheek, loving your enemies, looking within for more willingness and/or more humility. Whatever it takes to become the owner of your pain is what you do.

Acceptance is a gate through which one must pass on the way to dealing with emotional pain. If you don't pass through this gate, that is, if you are unable to claim ownership of your emotional pain, then it is not possible to deal with your pain in a successful manner. Once you own your pain you can be helped and can practice self-help. The following is a test to see if one has achieved acceptance: Ask yourself who is at fault for how you feel. If the answer is clearly yourself, someone else, or something else, then you are still into blame. Start over.

The above is a little bit general, but if you follow the steps, you are likely to find that you are a lot more competent to deal with emotional pain than you thought you were. It is also important that you eliminate from your vocabulary the word *can't*. Can't is simply a statement of unwillingness. There may be some things that we should be unwilling to do, but in matters of life management, willingness is usually much more effective than unwillingness.

The program for building life management skills which we use in our practice is based pretty much on the twelve step program that you may know as the basis for the Alcoholics Anonymous program. It is also used by Narcotics Anonymous, Emotions Anonymous, Overeaters Anonymous, and Parents Anonymous. It is best embodied in the Serenity Prayer:

> God, grant me the serenity to accept the things I cannot change, courage to change the things I can, and wisdom to know the difference.

SPIRITUAL HEALTH

An important part of the twelve step program, as well as a good life management program, is a way to achieve spiritual health. It is a clear need for the human condition and for one's own self-management. If you know about this and have a spiritual advisor, then you are in a good position to manage your own life. If this is unfamiliar territory, then you could obtain some practical information from a clergyman who works with alcoholics and who has given what is called the "fifth step." The fourth and fifth steps of the twelve step program are the spiritual component. It is understandable to almost anyone, and it will not interfere with one's own religion.

The fourth step of AA reads like this: "Made a searching and fearless moral inventory of ourselves." It is hard to embellish on these words, but others might call this process the examination of conscience. The fifth step is as follows: "Admitted to God, to ourselves, and to another human being the exact nature of our wrongs." A clergyman or some other spiritual advisor participates in the fifth step. It is much like the Sacrament of Confession in the Catholic Church. The reader is referred to the book *Alcoholics Anonymous*, [1] which is simple, practical, and easy to read.

A FAMILY ILLNESS

The problems of aging and the decreasing self-care ability in one family member is a family illness. All illnesses are family illnesses because they do affect the family dynamics of the entire system. If one person is sick the whole family is affected. Someone may assume a role previously held by the sick person. Someone else may not be able to complete a certain task without the help of the sick person. Everyone has a change of responsibility, and everyone feels some type of emotional pain. In some cases, an illness can have a severe impact on the family, and the family as a whole becomes so dysfunctional that it becomes the object of health care services. An example of this would be a family with Alzheimer's Disease where the spouse who is the primary caregiver is falling apart and unwilling to accept help.

A family meeting is suggested in order to bring everyone into the health care partnership. It is not good for the family to have one family member assume all of the responsibility. We can't afford to have caregivers with inadequate support, and we can't afford to have martyrs gumming up the family dynamics. It is good for people to help one another, and all problems are really an invitation and an opportunity for personal growth. No one should be protected from this opportunity for improving their own life management skills.

ESTABLISHING THE PARTNERSHIP

You are about to enter a relationship that requires the skills of a marriage and may involve more commitment and more intimacy than most marriages. Your health and the health of an elderly parent are at stake. I think you will want to choose carefully.

First of all, your partner needs to be someone who listens and who cares. If you have someone that you know and wish to consider, these are the criteria by which to judge. If you are shopping for the doctor, then consciously use these criteria as you make your decision. Do not settle for something less. You want a good relationship. You have learned through self-care how to be a good partner and now you must expect it in the other partner.

CHOOSING A PARTNER

I would tend to recommend a generalist as your personal physician and I have a preference for a family physician. This is because a family physician is exposed to the medical, social, environmental, and family factors in his everyday professional life. This kind of doctor is more aware of the needs of people and is willing to take the responsibility for both patients and their families. Board certified family physicians have an incentive to keep up to date because they are retested for certification at seven-year intervals. Another thing that appeals to me is that this type of physician is more willing to consult with other physicians because that is something he generally does on a regular basis.

If you have truly learned the lessons of self-management and self-care, then you may be more capable of partnership than the doctor you choose, but don't decide for the doctor that he isn't capable of partnership, because you will only end up creating a self-fulfilling prophecy. If you manage well, the doctor can learn from you. If you manage well and the doctor is unwilling to manage himself, then you are still okay and can look elsewhere. Remember that in general, if *you* practice self-manangement it is easier to ask it of others.

When it comes to partnership, don't be intimidated. Don't be hostile, but don't be put off. It will help to listen to and care about the physician with whom you are trying to establish a relationship.

Ask any questions that you want. If your emotional pain is well managed, then questions will come out of your good judgment. You want an advocate, a defender, a teacher, and someone who can help you negotiate through the health care system. If the things we have said thus far make sense to you and you can put them to use, then I would be able to write you a letter of recommendation, as follows:

Dear Doctor:

This letter will introduce a person who wishes to have your help and assistance in caring for her parents. She believes you are a person who will listen and who will care. She knows that she must contribute the ingredient of trust.

This is a person who may feel strongly and sometimes may even be overwhelmed by her own frustration or fear. She is not likely to take these feelings out on you because she has learned to accept and deal with her own emotional pain. She may need help in doing this but will not expect you to do it for her.

This is a difficult situation, and she needs your support. She would like to share in decision-making, be told what is going on, have your help in negotiating through the health care system, have you recommend second opinion or consultation where you think it would help, and have your guidance and direction as to how she can best carry out her own therapeutic role. In short, she would like to be in an adult collaborative relationship that is helpful to her, to you, and to the parent she wishes to care for.

I recommend this person to you as someone who knows how to be cooperative, collaborative, and negotiable. She is the kind of patient who you will find satisfying to your professional life because she can contribute to a good outcome. I wish you both well.

Signed,

A Family Physician and Friend of the Family

MAINTAINING THE PARTNERSHIP

PARTNERSHIP CONFLICT

Since the quality of the relationship will determine the quality of the outcome, it is clear that conflict should be avoided and dealt with rapidly if it should occur. First, decide that partnerships are too important to be thinking that dissolution is the answer. Tell yourself you are willing to clear the air and return to a good working relationship.

Think of things you can suggest such as: a third person arbiter, a second medical opinion, each person writing a list of their expectations, listening to each other (each listen for five minutes without interruption), ask for a clergyman of his choice or yours, or work on a contract that spells out how you want each other to behave.

I have acted as an intermediary to explain the risks of cardiac surgery or to explain to a family why the psychiatrist is recommending electro-convulsive therapy (ECT). I have helped patients of our practice resolve personal or financial conflicts with one of our consultants. One time a patient took something of mine and wouldn't give it back until I acquiesced to her demand. I wouldn't respond to her demand until she gave it back. Eventually we needed a third person to help us renegotiate our relationship.

Partnership Research

We have researched the partnership method and found that it has contributed significantly to the lives of our patients, and in some instances patients have credited it with saving their lives.

Through a grant from the National Institute of Child Health and Human Development (NICHD), our medical practice was able to evaluate its methods. Since we have a strong belief in the partnership method, we asked our patients to collaborate on the research.

Ten patients were selected who had serious life management problems such as suicidal depression, panic disorder, chemical dependency, or multiple medical problems. Each of those selected had moved from a losing lifestyle to a success-ful lifestyle using our program of health education. Focused group discussions between doctor and patients were used in the research, observed by the research professionals sitting outside the group.

These patients told us that they could provide the trust when the practitioners could provide listening and caring. Trust led to willingness, and willingness led to better participation in the process and improved information exchange, which in turn led to the development of life management skills. These skills empowered individuals to take responsibility and control of their lives.

These patients also said that it was necessary for practitioners to treat patients in a holistic way, to provide continuity of care over time, to speak in a language that is understandable and as simple as possible, and to focus on families as well as individual patients. At least three people in this particular group said that they owed their lives to the partnership process.

The Patient Advisory Council

The Patient Advisory Council is an idea that has been well tested and worked out in our medical practice over a fourteen-year period of time. The council provides the vehicle for a health care partnership between the practice staff and the patient group. It can solve some difficult problems, improve the management of the practice, and decrease the malpractice insurance premium. It is an organization that is protective of both doctors and patients.

The Patient Advisory Council is a formal relationship between the medical practice staff and the patient group. Its mission statement is as follows:

> A Patient Advisory Council is a medical practice advocate group made up of patients and health care professionals. They consult together to provide superior health care and services in a cost-effective manner while preserving the personal nature of the practitioner/patient relationship.

The council has a number of standing committees. They are as follows:

A. Organization
   1. *Membership Committee:* in charge of membership recruitment, reminding patients of meetings, soliciting comments, and mailing our various handouts
   2. *Treasury Committee:* the management of funds and paying of PAC bills, meeting arrangements (makes arrangements for place to hold meetings)
   3. *Recording Secretary:* takes the minutes and puts them in final form
B. Accountability
   1. *Policy Development and Assessment Committee:* reviews established policy, suggests revision, or requests new policy
   2. *Services Improvement Committee:* receives complaints, searches out actual circumstances, and gives useful criticism to the PAC and practice
   3. *Support Services Committee:* primarily involved with the business and financial aspects of practice management. The Accountability Committees need members with a strong interest in medical care delivery issues and problems. Business management experience and sensitivity to patient and physician needs are equally important for members of these committees
C. *Patient Services Committee:* takes responsibility for nonprofessional volunteer services to patients by patients, including the Talent Bank Registry and organization of community health education programs
D. *Liaison Committee:* makes and maintains contact with other PACs and is responsible for public relations generally for the PAC
E. *Research Committee:* develops, carries out and reports on projects to assess and improve health care delivery, such as patient satisfaction surveys

When someone writes me a nasty letter (usually refusing to pay their bill at the same time), I simply ask the Services Improvement Committee to look into the matter. Sometimes, the patient is way off base, and other times the patients return with recommendations to improve the practice services.

We have used members of the Talent Bank Committee to provide additional support and skills where necessary and where they are not otherwise available. Such services would include homemaking, babysitting, transportation, and shopping. Our patients like to do these things and in a couple of instances have made home care possible where it otherwise would not have been.

Businessmen have joined in business management and have contributed good ideas which have led to a more efficient medical practice. However, it is the idea of partnership and the ability to resolve patient complaints that has prompted our malpractice insurance carrier to give us a 10 percent discount. If you were to ask them, they would say that they believe these practices lead to safer patient care.

You might want to approach your own physician with the idea that he begin a Patient Advisory Council or that he let you see if you can organize a group of his patients. There are several advantages to the physician and the practice, and the possibility of reducing the medical malpractice premium is a real incentive.

REFERENCE

1. *Alcoholics Anonymous*. (New York: AA World Services, 1976).

RECOMMENDED READINGS

Barnard, P. "Comfort and Medical Care," *The Journal of Family Practice* 23 (1986):495–96.
Cohen, H. *You Can Negotiate Anything*. Secaucus, N.J.: Lyle Stuart, 1980.
Peck, S. M. *The Road Less Traveled*. New York: Simon & Schuster, 1978.
Starting Your Own Patient Advisory Council, available from: MD Publishing Company, Box 363, Spring Park, MN 55384.

Forgiving

the Reverend Tanya Vonnegut Beck

Of all the inner transactions, forgiveness may be the most difficult. It means letting go, taking new risks, and sometimes forcing painful confrontations with yourself and with others. At points of crisis in the caregiving role—finding ourselves faced with old unfinished business, resolving conflicts, struggling to get through our parents' final days (even at the funeral old hurts and tensions often erupt in anger), discovering that we may even feel angry toward the loved one who left us—we may feel the need to be forgiven, or to forgive.

In traveling around the country in the last ten to twelve years talking to many people in many places, I have found that the issue of forgiveness is one element in our lives that is misunderstood, mistaken, and is one that we need to understand and use more meaningfully. The act of forgiveness, forgiveness of ourselves and forgiveness of other people, is a very difficult act to perform. It is not easy to truly forgive. To forgive is to understand wrong, to release emotions, and to be ready to risk again; that asks a great deal of us. Forgiveness, however, is the core of the deepest, most fulfilling, most meaningful, most giving kind of love. We must face the fact that in our humanness real, honest, forgiveness is difficult, very difficult, but not impossible. Most negative relational situations,

The Reverend Tanya Vonnegut Beck, founder and director of the Julian Center, Indianapolis, Indiana, has served with three parishes of the Episcopal Diocese. As a middle school teacher she has designed special programs to meet the needs of the economically and physically disabled. She is owner/manager of her own business, Communicators, Inc.

207

we tolerate. We don't truly forgive. It is ludicrous to lightly throw the term around; however, we say it all the time. I laughingly will say, "Oh, I forgive you, don't worry about it. I forgive you." When I say that, I really mean I accept the reality of the wrongdoing. I accept releasing my fear, my anger, my ego needs around the act, and I cancel my demand that you change. I work through the levels of anger and pain challenging them over and over until the ability to risk and trust emerge. I resist demanding an iron-clad guarantee that the behavior will not occur again, and I accept the possibility of failure with you again and again and again. So you see, forgiveness is not to be taken lightly. Forgiveness is an act of passion, equally as important in the balance of life as love, faith, and hope. Actually it's the integral element present in all three that enables us to go on to growth, to change, to inner peace.

What are the elements in the act of forgiving? The first element is time. You cannot hurry to really forgive. Space is second. Do not crowd to really forgive. Third, there must be the willingness to see another's word and acts as genuinely repentant, genuinely sorry. Fourth, you must be willing to trust the other by risking being wronged again. Fifth, you must be willing to be open to relate again in wholesome ways. Sixth, you must be willing to venture into new closeness.

Forgiving goes two ways. Forgiving means to forgive another and to receive forgiveness. The elements involved in receiving forgiveness are the same in the beginning—lots of time is needed for each party to ascertain that their feelings have settled down enough to begin to receive the forgiveness. Space is needed—space apart, space giving air and room to grow to the point where you are willing and able to receive the forgiveness. There must be a willingness to affirm the sorrow—to trust my own responses and to risk freely again. To be open again with both candor and caring and to be close to you without fear. How close we can become to the person we have hurt or who hurt us so deeply is often times a matter of degree in the reality of life. I think we have to be real and accept that. To honestly forgive another means to honestly accept our own limitations—limitations such as our fear of aloneness, of abandonment, of rejection, our sense of powerlessness at times. We must accept those feelings within us in order for us to understand why others have reacted in the desperate way they have toward us. Only then can we understand the roots of the issues facing those to be forgiven.

For most acts of wrongdoing that need forgiveness are connected to poor self-image. We feel so "lousy" about ourselves that we want, unconsciously or consciously, to make others miserable. To honestly forgive and be forgiven means giving up the following attitudes:

>   blaming—"Well, it's all your fault."
>   avoidance—"I don't want to talk about it."

magical ritual—"I'm so sorry."
denial—"Problem! What problem? I don't have a problem."
displacement—"Have you heard the latest?"
undoing—"I'll make it up to you."

All these are powerless and useless in restoring relationships. They don't fit true forgiveness. Two of the skills we need in order to understand and activate true forgiveness are the skill of letting go and the skill of confronting. Letting go specifically means letting go of grudges. Letting go of the past. Letting go of the history. Holding on to resentments and grudges results in the following kinds of manifestation: I demand that you turn time back and undo what is already done. In other words, change it for me. Take it away. Make it a different way. Second, I demand that you change the unchangeable. Do it! Don't talk to me. Do it! Third, I demand you appease, pacify, grovel, suffer in atonement for your inability to do the impossible, which is to respond to me the way that I want you to. Seldom can that occur. I'm holding in and holding on, and when that occurs no change, no growth is possible to us. So holding on to resentments is a very negative approach to the act of forgiveness. Letting go is the important issue here. I hold grudges because it is safe to do that. If I let go of the grudge, I must release the pain, and then I must confront. And confronting may risk my power level because you see, if I hold the grudge, I've got a lot of power over you. If I let go of the grudge, then the pain all comes up to the top, and then I have to say to you, "What can we do? I feel terrible."

Confrontation almost always lowers our "threat" level, though. It makes us more vulnerable, but when we lower our threat level we become more equal in the engagement of one human being to another. When we meet each other on more equal terms, we feel less manipulated, less persecuted. When we feel able to stand on our own, less persecuted, we can confront wrongdoings and let go of the grudgeful feelings, and when that happens then the process of accepting can begin.

The process of forgiveness looks something like this:

1. Seeing the other as having worth again regardless of the wrongdoing. Seeing that human being as a worthwhile, unique, beautiful person even though he or she is limited.
2. Seeing the other as equally precious again in spite of the pain we are feeling. Seeing the other person in deep pain, and although we feel alienated from them, understanding that they are a very precious human being who has in all their humanness made an error that has affected our lives. And in the midst of the pain, accepting that reality.
3. Cancelling the demands of the past. Recognizing that changing the unchange-able is impossible and accepting the reality of the present.

4. Working through the anger and the pain felt by both in reciprocal trusting and risking until genuineness is perceived by both people.

5. Dropping the demands for an iron-clad guarantee of future behavior—and opening the future to choice, to spontaneity, and then of course to the possibility of failing again. And being present with that person if failure occurs.

6. Touching each other deeply. Feeling moved—warmth, love, and compassion. Celebrating it in mutual recognition that right relationships have been achieved. Now the right relationship may be no relationship at all except perhaps the acknowledgment of a friendship. The mutual recognition may be that that person is no longer available for the kind of relationship you had with them in the past.

The bottom line of forgiveness is self-acceptance and self-care. If you choose to feel guilty all the rest of your life, you choose to stop growing, really living. If you choose to forgive yourself, you choose to cope with life, to grope, to keep struggling, to find new behaviors that will serve you in a more positive manner. Remember that forgiveness requires time, space, releasing grudges, confrontation, and a good sense of self-worth—a passion for life.

Now, in looking at this very serious subject, what aspects do you need to work on in the business of forgiveness of self and others? It might be helpful to you to ask these questions:

1. Who still needs the forgiveness in a particular situation? You or the other person?

2. What risks are you afraid of in this forgiving act? Are you afraid of more rejection? Of seeming foolish? Of being vulnerable again?

3. What action steps must you take to get yourself ready to confront openly?

4. What anger or persecuted feelings are you hanging on to, and what need are those feelings filling for you?

5. What support do you need in order to face the pain of forgiveness? And where can you receive that support?

6. What new feelings of release and freedom can you imagine as you enter into the act of true forgiveness?

In closing, I would just like to say this—it has been my experience that it is far easier to forgive others than to forgive ourselves. We sometimes wallow in guilt. We are afraid to give up guilt because even if we don't like it, we do understand it. We know it. For some of us it's a very good friend. It seems far more risky and insecure to let go of the guilt and honestly forgive ourselves and move on into new behavior. I recently was confronting that very issue with myself. I realized that I had forgiven the person with whom I had had a very difficult relationship some three years ago. I'd long ago forgiven that person, but I still hadn't forgiven myself. And I had to look at *why*. It came down to some pretty basic things. I wasn't really ready to risk a new relationship yet. I wasn't sure that I wanted to take on the responsibility of being an earnest seeker for relationships again. I was scared.

And so, take a look at your life. What's holding you back from forgiving yourself? Try loving yourself enough to forgive yourself. To give yourself the honest opportunity to move forward with a passion for life in a positive, forgiving manner.

Notes on Support
and Resources

Jane Norris

"I felt a sense of relief when I first encountered other women who are confronted with problems identical to my own."

"I live in a world of love and joy, misery and pain. It's good to share it with others."

These are daughters' comments quoted in the support group brochure. "I am alone" is often one of the first messages we hear from daughters who attend the meetings. It is because of this sense of isolation that we have wanted, through this book, to come as close as we could to sharing the support of the group with you. And it is our hope that you

are more encouraged to take care of yourself,
have a stronger sense of autonomy,
feel a little better about your feelings,
believe that you *can* find support and the partners that you need,
have added somewhat to your skills in and knowledge about caregiving,
and have talked some of it over with your family.

This is in large part what the group members themselves have worked on in the weekly meetings for seven years. On these final pages I have some thoughts—notes, so to speak—on support and resources.

Jane Norris, BSN, RN, has held staff and faculty positions in hospitals, a doctor's office, a student health center, a nursing home, schools of nursing, and a mental health center. Jane and her husband, Dick, are finally settled (in a long-awaited country home) with their daughter and sons and grandchildren nearby.

212

ON SUPPORT

Support . . . when we're tired, and often when we need it the most, seems to be the hardest time to find it. I think that is because we often wait until we're *too* desperate. Perhaps the other, the husband, the children, the professional, would not retreat in confusion if we were able to explain a little more calmly (or rationally, some might say) what it is that we are seeking. That involves a little homework on our parts, and it is a difficult task because it involves allowing ourselves the "luxury" of stopping a little while to get our thoughts in order. It involves identifying the problems, deciding which ones take priority right at this moment and which ones someone else can realistically help us with, and then not allowing our feelings to get in the way of working it out with the other person, the partner, whoever that may be. Again, this is not an easy task for worn-out caregivers who are pressed for time. This is one of the ways a support group can be helpful. While it's true that groups don't work for everyone (perhaps quiet reflection or talking to a friend or professional helps), it's also true that a group of caring people who face similar situations can provide a great deal for each other in a comfortable setting on a regular basis.

If you'd like to try a support group and there is not one available, you might think about starting one. Work through a network you already know—a church, a neighborhood association, or a local agency. You may find others ready and eager to participate, to learn, and to share with you. The three areas that are the most sought-after in the caregiving role are education, support, and respite. A group can offer all three to some degree. In the early days of DEBUT we offered many educational programs—over thirty before the end of the second year—based specifically on the needs of the current members. The programs were usually films, tapes, or presentations by people in the community. We found that it was not advisable to offer educational programs on a weekly basis because members needed support, needed to talk with each other, sometimes even before *one* week had passed! The members have always stressed confidentiality and that support be *non*-judgmental support, as one person's solution may not be the one that works for another. Attending the meetings provides some amount of respite, and members share with each other ways in which they have been able to obtain some time for self-renewal.

After I had spent several months with the group, I realized that all of us (women, daughters, caregivers) at one time or another have difficulty identifying ourselves—to others and even to ourselves—within the context of the caregiving role. So I wrote the following mock "history and physical." I wrote it for the fun of it but also with an awareness of the seriousness of the total picture of the daughter, with an awareness that we cannot always see our own picture or describe it to someone else. I hope you enjoy it; it was meant to be humorous. I hope you take it seriously; it is a composite of many very real daughters. Although it is no one daughter, every caregiving daughter may be able to find herself in here somewhere. If you have had trouble expressing this to your doctor, if you are afraid his impression might be "tired housewife syndrome," or some other such diagnosis, try talking this over with him; perhaps together you can find "you."

Daughter's History and Physical

Patient: Caregiving Daughter
Age: 35–70+
Address: Everywhere, USA
Number: Almost Up

Chief Complaint: "I can't go on any longer. I'm doing this alone."

Presenting Problem: Fatigue, general malaise, emotional trauma, disruption of nuclear family, bouts of depression. Assaulted by strong feelings of frustration, inadequacy, anger, fear, guilt, helplessness, hopelessness, perceived isolation, and sadness. Despairs over need for practical information.

History: Father deceased. Mother, living, but not well. Mother suffers from diabetes, osteoarthritis, and angina. Has turned to daughter for support and assistance, but at the same time is resistent to any change which is not compatible with her self-image and former lifestyle. Daughter is visiting mother daily, seeking sound medical, psycho-social advice, providing wide range of supports to mother, working outside the home, meeting the demands of roles as wife and mother, and beginning to experience age-related transitions herself.

Physical: All systems appear within normal limits. However, on closer examination, immune system manifests red-alert overload, and all reserves for homeostasis are on verge of bankruptcy.

Impression: Technical information deficiency
Atrophy of reserves
Recurrent isolation syndrome
Pernicious emotional hemophilia

Treatment Plan: Nourish with information about aging, aged-related disorders
Exercise permission and skills for taking care of self
Administer broad-spectrum resources
Transfuse empathic dose of "peer expert" support and counseling

Prognosis: Until this daughter finds the support, education, and respite needed to carry out the tasks expected of her, by her own standards and others, prognosis remains poor, for her and for *her* daughter.

ON RESOURCES

Do not be intimidated by what you don't know. What you need is out there somewhere. Reach out. Even though it's difficult to do, even if you've never had to do it before, reach out to someone for what you need.

If you don't know where to take that first step, perhaps the reference librarian at the library could help you locate some material that would point you in the right direction. If you reach out and are thwarted for some reason, don't stop there. Find another name, make another call, get another opinion; at some point, you will recognize what feels right.

The task, the multiple tasks, of caregiving can be overwhelming. But it's getting better. With growing awareness of the increasing population of the elderly and their increasing needs, health care providers and members of the helping professions are also reaching out as partners to the elderly and to their caregivers.

I want to share with you a letter which came to us in 1983. We often refer to it, "Wendi's letter," with joy (because Wendi wrote to us and we were able to correspond with her) and with concern (because it made us even more aware of the intergenerational impact of today's "aging"). Wendi is a thirteen-year-old girl who reached out to us across several hundred miles because of concern for her mother and her family.

Wendi wrote to us again about a year later. This time her letter was typed. She ended by saying:

> It's hard to bear the thought of putting my grandmother in an institution. I don't think that is the answer, but I don't know what is. My mom hates the idea too; after all, it is her mother. And my grandmother is still able to take care of herself with most things.
>
> I love my grandmother but I love my mother much more and if it is going to cause her physical problems and mental stress to the point where she feels batty herself—I just don't know. There is a point where she has to stop and see what it is doing to herself. She'll go nuts.
>
> Mom sent for some of the books in your bibliography and all of us are thankful for the information you sent.
>
> God bless you ever so much,
> Wendi

When you think about resources, don't forget to put your parent at the top of the list. Identification of physical, mental, and emotional condition is a first step in determining which direction to go. Assessment—understanding whether or not what you see has a physical, mental, or emotional cause—is vital to the decisions you and your parent will make. Professionals can help you especially with determinations in the first two areas. Perhaps you and your parent together can make accurate assessments in the emotional area, as you know your parent more personally and his or her situation better than the professionals will. It will

Wendi

DEBUT
% Jane Norris
Bloomington, Indiana

Dear Ladies:

We sure need help I saw your an article about your group in my grandmother's ~~morally~~ ~~Theodore~~ Maturity. My mom is 41 o, she has my sister and I to deal with, and my grandmother (her mother, lives with us and is slipping. The living-with-the family-bit is just till we can get up a house for her and one for us. We are living in a 24 ft. travel trailer. There is no privacy and that is wearing since mom and dad like to talk and Lisa, my older sister -14-, and I, 13, like privacy too. The is no Real remedy for that, but can you pleas send an address to correspond to and some information. We all love Gran and its awful. You see our other grandparents are going a little slippy to, but - thanks heavens - they live 500 mi away.

Thank you!

P.S. Please send info to my mother her address an

be very important for you and your parent, however, to pass this understanding of your parent's feeling and situation along to the professional helpers. It will help them to know if your parent is grieving, or lonely, or frustrated and angry.

Nursing homes are one of our resources, and as Lisa says, "institutional options will not go away—nor should they." It is very likely that you or I or both of us will be residents in a nursing home at some time, even if only for a short stay. I believe that we can make nursing homes part of the community—that *we* can reach out to *them* for the improvements, the care, that we seek. We can serve (with training) as volunteers (we do in hospitals), as visitors to the residents, as leaders in establishing more closely the community we seek within the nursing home. We can work with the staff and administration of nursing homes to get where *we* want to be.

Resources or agencies have been mentioned throughout the book. Locally you will want to find a way to enter into the "aging network." If you don't know someone personally who can offer suggestions for what you need, or if you can't find resources through the physician or the hospital, you might try contacting, or visiting, a local Older Americans Center. There someone might be able to refer you to an agency for the information you seek, such as a Public Health Nursing Office, a Visiting Nurse Service, the County Health Department, or a Family Services Agency. Most areas have available a Community Mental Health Center; although many of these do not have specialized geriatric teams they may have services to help you, or might be able to refer you. Also, most areas have available an Area Agency, or Council, on Aging where they provide assistance and services to the elderly. Whether you're seeking information, support, or respite, as in an adult day care program or home health care, many of these agencies (sometimes listed in special sections in the telephone book) will be able to help you, or refer you. It frequently takes some detective work and persistence, but eventually you will find what you and your parent need. It will be most helpful to you if you start this process of becoming part of the network before you and your family are faced with a crisis.

There are times when what we need, what is just right for us, is not a part of the traditional scene or network. These are the times to search for different solutions. I want to offer an example and finish on that, more personal, note.

I too, until recently, was a daughter of the elderly, and am now, as Glen Davidson says, an orphan. My two brothers and I were long-distance caregivers to our mother who was still living alone in her home but declining from dementia, although like others, it took us awhile to comprehend it. It became apparent when we visited, when we learned that she had driven thirty miles in the wrong direction to visit one of us, when the neighbors told us of an evening walk in the rain, that it was becoming dangerous for her to continue to live in the country home she loved. So, we too went through the long process: phone calls, worrying with each other long distance; wondering what we could do; agonizing over what we could not do; and searching for answers and help. Guardianship seemed necessary to Mother's care, so we gathered together in her home, and she signed the papers—not a joyous occasion, as you can imagine, but as I said, it allowed us to provide for her care.

We had to decide what to do. I remembered spending a week with her earlier that year and knew that I could not personally, emotionally, take care of her. I remembered one ten-minute period in which she first said to me, "I remember when we used to play together," and then minutes later said, "I used to be a teacher, and look at me now." By the end of the week I was lying on the couch and Mom was covering *me* with an afghan.

Because Mom loved to be in the country, because she loved to have animals near her, we looked for alternatives. We decided on a private caregiving home in a country setting with vegetable gardens and flowers, children, and kittens and puppies.

Any of you who have experienced visiting a demented parent will know how much I appreciated the wonderful lady who was Mom's caregiver, and who wrote the following note to you. She met me at the door with hugs, and giving me a peck on the cheek as I left each time, said, "Don't worry, Janie, I know how hard it is."

The idea of home care came to my sister and me during the time our father became ill and needed constant supervision at the early age of fifty-five. Dad needed someone with him day and night and good reliable live-in help is very hard to come by, not to mention expensive. The only option we had at the time was a nursing home since we both worked and had small children. Dad had good care in the nursing home, but there was something missing. Our father was a very loving and outgoing person, and he loved having his family and friends around. Dad seemed to change and became more withdrawn and moody after several months in the nursing home. He was receiving good care and his physical needs were being met, but the emotional ones were not. It is very difficult, or impossible, to have a one-to-one relationship with your patients when you work in a nursing home no matter how hard you try. There's just not enough time or help.

Even after Dad passed away the idea of home care stayed at the back of our minds. By then Sis and I had left our other jobs. We were taking care of a lady in her home, each doing a twelve-hour shift, when the family decided that they could no longer keep up the expense of a home and twenty-four-hour-a-day care for her. We talked it over with our families and then discussed the idea of home care with her family. They thought it was a great idea, so since Sis had just remodeled her home and had a private room with bath, she took the lady home with her, and I went to work for her three days a week. A few months later I was working with her full time; two other ladies had joined the first, referred by word of mouth. (Our best form of advertising comes from the families and friends of the elderly who live with us.) The State Board of Health has supervised us, and we are allowed, in home care, to have three residents.

We share the work and responsibilities, including trips to the doctor's office, the beauty salon, and family outings; one person cannot do this on her own. For us it is a family project. We all work and we all benefit. Our children bring joy to the elderly and they in turn give a fuller understanding of life to our kids. I know our children are more compassionate and understanding because of their contact with "our" elderly people.

In order to do a good job with this kind of service you need to have a true love for elderly people. They need someone who is loving (kisses *can* cure), understanding yet firm, compassionate, and patient. Our people become part of our lives, and we become part of theirs. Therefore, it is very important that we have the support of their families, friends, and doctors.

If you are thinking about this kind of service you can contact several sources for information: (*a*) doctors and ministers, (*b*) Public Health Nursing, (*c*) hospital patient referral, (*d*) Mental Health agencies (for aged), or (*e*) any service that works with the elderly, such as Area Agencies on Aging.

The family doctor is a good source of information and very helpful to us. We do not provide medical care. We do work with the doctors and follow their orders the same as we would with our own families. In short, what we provide for our elderly people is a home environment. We cook, clean, listen, love, and watch after them just as if they were our own. We try to give them a feeling of usefulness and belonging. After all, that is what life is all about.

BIBLIOGRAPHY

ADULT CHILDREN AND PARENTS

Bloomfield, Harold H., with Leonard Felder. *Making Peace with Your Parents.* New York: Random House, 1983.

Brubacker, T. H., and D. Springer. *Family Caregivers and Dependent Elderly.* Beverly Hills, CA: Sage Publications, 1985.

Bumagin, Victoria E., and Kathryn Hirn. *Aging Is a Family Affair.* New York: Thomas Y. Crowell, 1979.

Cohen, Stephen Z., and Bruce Michael Gans. *The Other Generation Gap: The Middle-aged and Their Aging Parents.* Chicago: Follett, 1978.

Halpern, Howard M. *Cutting Loose: A Guide to Adult Relationships with Your Parents.* New York: Simon & Schuster, 1977.

Horne, Jo. *Caregiving: Helping an Aged Loved One.* Washington, DC: American Association of Retired Persons, 1985.

Kenny, James, and Stephen Spicer. *Caring for Your Aging Parent: A Practical Guide to the Challenges, the Choices.* Cincinnati: St. Anthony Messenger Press, 1984.

Levy, Judith. *Grandmother Remembers.* New York: Stewart, Tabori & Chang, 1983.

Otten, J., and F. D. Shelley. *When Your Parents Grow Old.* New York: Funk & Wagnalls, 1976.

Silverstone, Barbara, and Helen Kandel Hyman. *You and Your Aging Parent: The Modern Family's Guide to Emotional, Physical, and Financial Problems.* Rev. and enl. ed. New York: Pantheon, 1982.

Smith, Bert Kruger. *The Pursuit of Dignity.* Boston: Beacon Press, 1977.

Somers, Tish, and Laurie Shields. *Women Take Care: The Consequences of Caregiving in Today's Society.* Gainesville, FL: Triad, 1987.

Stern, Edith M., and Mabel Ross. *You and Your Aging Parents.* New York: Harper and Row, 1965.

AGING

Blythe, Ronald. *View in Winter.* New York: Harcourt Brace Jovanovich, 1979.

Callahan, Daniel. *Setting Limits: Medical Goals in an Aging Society.* New York: Simon & Schuster, 1987.

Comfort, Alex. *A Good Age.* New York: Crown, 1976.

221

Kaufman, Sharon. *The Ageless Self: Sources of Meaning in Late Life*. Madison: University of Wisconsin Press, 1986.

Kornhaber, Arthur. *Grandparents and Grandchildren: The Vital Connection*. Garden City, NY: Anchor Press, 1981.

Stokell, Marjorie, and Bonnie Kennedy. *The Senior Citizen Handbook*. Englewood Cliffs, NJ: Prentice-Hall, 1985.

DEMENTIA

Cohen, Donna, and Carl Isdorfer. *The Loss of Self: A Family Resource for the Care of Alzheimer's Disease and Related Disorders*. New York: Norton, 1986.

Kra, Siegfried. *Aging Myths: Reversible Causes of Mind and Memory Loss*. New York: McGraw-Hill, 1986.

Mace, Nancy L., and Peter V. Rabins. *The 36-Hour Day*. Baltimore: The Johns Hopkins University Press, 1981.

McDowell, F. H., ed. *Managing the Person with Intellectual Loss (Dementia or Alzheimer's Disease) at Home*. White Plains, NY: Burke Rehabilitation Center, 1980.

Powell, Lenore S., and Katie Courtice. *Alzheimer's Disease: A Guide for Families*. Reading, MA: Addison-Wesley, 1983.

Zarit, Steven H., Nancy K. Orr, and Judy M. Zarit. *The Hidden Victims of Alzheimer's Disease*. New York: New York University Press, 1985.

HEALTH

Ardell, Donald B. *14 Days to a Wellness Lifestyle*. Mill Valley, CA: Whatever, 1982.

Briggs, Dorothy Corkille. *Celebrate Your Self*. Garden City, NY: Doubleday, 1977.

Budoff, Penny Wise. *No More Hot Flashes*. New York: G. P. Putnam's Sons, 1983.

Burns, David D. *Feeling Good: A New Mood Therapy*. New York: William Morrow, 1980.

Cohen, Donna, and Carl Eisdorfer. *The Loss of Self*. New York: W. W. Norton, 1986.

Conahan, Judith M. *Helping Your Elderly Patients: A Guide for Nursing Assistants*. New York: Tiresias Press, 1976.

Graedon, Joe. *The People's Pharmacy—2*. New York: Avon Books, 1980.

Haney, Michelle, and Edmond W. Boenisch. *Stress Map—Finding Your Pressure Points*. San Luis Obispo. CA: Impact, 1982.

Inlander, Charles B. *Take This Book to the Hospital with You*. Emmaus, PA: Rodale Press, 1985.

Bibliography

2 2 3 223

Bibliography223

Scarf, Maggie. *Unfinished Business: Pressure Points in the Lives of Women.* New York: Ballantine, 1980.

Selye, Hans. *Stress without Distress.* New York: Signet, 1974.

"Stand Tall: A Women's Guide to Preventing Osteoporosis." Triad Publications, P.O. Box 13096, Gainsville, Florida 32604.

Stern, Bert, and Lawrence D. Chilnick. *The Pill Book.* New York: Bantam Books, 1979.

HOUSING

Bennett, Clifford. *Nursing Home Life: What It Is and What It Could Be.* New York: Tiresias Press, 1980.

Gold, Margaret. *Guide to Housing Alternatives for Older Citizens.* Mount Vernon, NY: Consumer Reports Books, 1985.

Nassau, Jean Baron. *Choosing a Nursing Home.* New York: Funk & Wagnalls, 1975.

Raper, Ann Trublood. *National Continuing Care Directory.* Washington, DC: American Association of Retired Persons, 1984.

LOSS AND GRIEF

Beauvoir, Simone de. *A Very Easy Death.* New York: G. P. Putnam's Sons, 1966.

Bozarth-Campbell, Alla. *Life Is Goodbye, Life is Hello: Grieving Well through All Kinds of Loss.* Minneapolis: CompCare, 1982.

Davidson, Glen W. *Understanding Mourning.* Minneapolis: Augsburg, 1984.

Grollman, Earl A. (ed). *Concerning Death: A Practical Guide for the Living.* Boston: Beacon Press, 1974.

Kubler-Ross, Elisabeth. *On Death and Dying.* New York: Macmillan, 1969.

Kushner, Harold S. *When Bad Things Happen to Good People.* New York: Schocken Books, 1981.

Myers, Edward. *When Parents Die: A Guide for Adults.* New York: Viking Penguin, 1986.

O'Connor, Nancy. *Letting Go with Love: The Grieving Process.* Apache Junction, AZ: Mariposa Press, 1984.

Staudacher, Carol. *Beyond Grief: A Guide for Recovering from the Loss of a Loved One.* Oakland, CA: New Harbinger Publications, 1987.

Stearns, Ann Kaiser. *Living through Personal Crisis.* New York: Ballantine, 1984.